The Gen X S

MW00997584

MATHS
OLYMPIAD 4

Useful for Maths Olympiads Conducted at School, National & International Levels

Author
Shraddha Singh

Peer Reviewer
Nisha Dhiman

Strictly According to the Latest Syllabus of Maths Olympiad

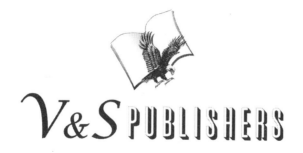

V&S PUBLISHERS

Published by:

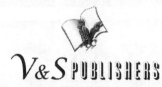

V&S PUBLISHERS

F-2/16, Ansari road, Daryaganj, New Delhi-110002
☎ 23240026, 23240027 • *Fax:* 011-23240028
✉ info@vspublishers.com • 🌐 www.vspublishers.com

 Online Brandstore: amazon.in/vspublishers

Regional Office : Hyderabad
5-1-707/1, Brij Bhawan (Beside Central Bank of India Lane)
Bank Street, Koti, Hyderabad - 500 095
☎ 040-24737290
✉ vspublishershyd@gmail.com

Follow us on:

BUY OUR BOOKS FROM: AMAZON FLIPKART

DISCLAIMER

Printed at : Param Offsetters, Okhla, New Delhi–110020

Publisher's Note

The current decade has firmly established V&S Publishers as one of the Leading Publishers of General Trade Mass Appeal Books across popular genres along with Academic Books for school children. Having been in publishing trade for over 40 years we understand the need of the hour when it comes to Books. After successfully publishing over 600 titles in a rather short time span of 5 years and establishing a pan India network of booksellers & distributors including ecommerce platforms viz – Amazon, Flipkart etc; an extensive market research lead us to publishing our Bestselling Series ever – OLYMPIAD BOOKS.

The Olympiad Series launched 4 years back under our GEN X SERIES Imprint gained widespread popularity amongst students and teachers immediately owing to its rich, high quality content and unique presentation. Published for Classes 1–10 across subjects English, Maths, Science & Computers, these books are holistic in nature and unlike run of the mill workbooks in the market, which are mere replicas of one another, these books deal with the content in a much comprehensive manner. Recourse to the 'Principles of Applied Psychology of Student Learning' has been utilised to upgrade levels of conceptual understanding in all designated subjects among class 1 to 10 students.

Encouraged by this huge acceptability of our Olympiad Series among parents and students and after revolutionising the way Olympiad books were written and published, we at V&S Publishers decided to take this to the next level.

We present to you Brand New Edition of our book – **MATHS OLYMPIAD CLASS 4.**

Each book originally written by Subject Matter Expert, is now further Peer Reviewed by top School Teachers and HODs to eliminate the slightest of errors that were present earlier. Furthermore to ensure authenticity and accuracy of content the book is now completely revised and reformatted as per the guidelines of the examining body. The New and Revised Olympiad Book is now suited to Olympiad examinations conducted at School Level, National Level or International Level by any and all organisations/companies.

The New Edition of this Maths Olympiad Class 4 is written in a Guide like pattern with images and illustrations at every step & is divided into different sections. Each chapter comes with Basic Theory and Solved Examples. Multiple Choice Questions with their Answer Keys and Solutions are liberally included. In order to help students become aware of and to simulate the actual exam conditions, a bunch of OMR Sheets have been enclosed with the book as well.

Amalgamation of Technology with Content has always been at the forefront for V&S Publishers and our new Student Portal for Olympiad Practice–www.vsexamprep.com is further testimony to that. We recommend students logging in and using it to their benefit.

P.S. While every care has been taken to ensure correctness of content, if you come across any error, howsoever minor, anywhere in the book, do not hesitate to discuss with your teachers while pointing that out to us in no uncertain terms.

We wish you All The Best!

Contents

Contents

SECTION 1
MATHEMATICAL REASONING

Number System

> **Learning Objectives**
> In this chapter, students will learn about:
> - Numbers (Numerals) and Number Names
> - 5-digit and 6-digit Numbers
> - Place Value and Face Value
> - Comparing Numbers
> - Successor and Predecessor
> - Ascending and Descending Order
> - Even and Odd Number
> - Expanded Form of Numbers
> - Forming Numbers
> - Rounding Numbers

Numbers (Numerals)

We use numbers in each and every sphere of our life. Large numbers are often used in monetary transactions in businesses, banks, etc. Total number of schools in a city, total number of students in a university are all examples of large numbers.

Number Names

Let us have a look at the table given below:

Number	Number Name
1	One
10	Ten
100	One hundred
1000	One thousand
10000	Ten thousand
100000	One lakh
1000000	Ten lakh

Numbers shown in the table are based on Indian System of numeration. As the number increases, it becomes larger and larger.

As we know there are ten digits: 0, 1, 2, 3, 4, 5, 6, 7, 8 and 9. Numbers are written using these digits. These digits are called ones. The numerals formed by the digits 0, 1, 2, 3, 4, ... are known as Hindu-Arabic numbers. This system is popular world-wide.

Numeral system is a way of counting and naming number. Number is an idea whereas the symbols used to represent the numbers are called numerals.

5-digit Numbers

9999 is the largest 4-digit number. If we add 1 to it, it will give us the smallest 5-digit number.

6-digit Numbers

We know that 99,999 is the greatest 5-digit number. If we add 1 to it, it will give us the smallest 6-digit number.

Place Value

Place value of a digit depends on its position in the number. As the digit moves to the left, its value increases. The face value of a digit in a number is the value of digit itself.

Indian Number System

Lakhs Period		Thousands Period		Ones Period		
Ten Lakhs (TL)	Lakhs (L)	Ten Thousands (TTh)	Thousands (Th)	Hundreds (H)	Tens (T)	Ones (O)

The place value chart has been separated into three groups: Ones period – It has three places: Hundreds, tens and ones. Thousands period – It has two places: Ten thousands and thousands.

Lakhs period – It has two places: Ten lakhs and lakhs.

Interntional Number System

Thousands period			Ones period		
Hundred Thousands (HTh)	Ten Thousands (TTh)	Thousands (TTh)	Hundreds (H)	Tens (T)	Ones (0)

Use of Commas

(i) If we write the number without using the place values chart, we use comma to separate the periods. Let us take an example: 4,57,283

(ii) In the Indian number system, first comma is used when the ones period is complete.

(iii) Second comma is used when thousands period is complete. Next comma is used to separate thousands and lakhs period.

(iv) In the International number system, put a comma after every three digits, starting from the right.

Comparing Numbers

The number which has more number of digits is greater.

For example, 855267 is greater than 28572.

(i) If two numbers have the same number of digits and the extreme left digits are also the same, then compare the next digits to the right and so on.

For example, 34291 is greater than 33203.

(ii) If two numbers have the same number of digits, then the number with bigger digit on the extreme left is greater. For example, 573235 is greater than 358496.

Successor and Predecessor

(i) The number that comes just after a given number is called its successor.

Example: Write the successor of the following numbers.

578, 284, 999

Solution:

Number	Successor
578	579
284	285
999	1000

(ii) The successor of a number is obtained by adding 1 to that number.

(iii) The number that comes just before a particular number is called its predecessor.

Example: Write the predecessor of the following numbers.

178, 195, 285

Solution:

Number	Predecessor
178	177
195	194
285	284

(iv) Clearly the predecessor of a number is obtained by subtracting 1 from the given number.

Note: Zero has no predecessor.

Ascending and Descending Order

Arranging the given numbers from the smallest to the greatest is called the ascending order or increasing order.

Example: Arrange the following numbers in ascending order.

4572, 5132, 4698, 8455

Solution: All the given numbers are 4-digit numbers. So, on comparing their thousands place we get, $4 < 5 < 8$

But thousands place of 4572 and 4698 are same. So on comparing their hundreds place we get,

$5 < 6$

$\Rightarrow 4572 < 4698$

Hence, $4572 < 4698 < 5132 < 8455$

$\therefore$ Ascending order is 4572, 4698, 5132, 8455

Arranging the given number from the greatest to the smallest is called the descending order or decreasing order.

Example: Arrange the following numbers in descending order.

5431, 3451, 5231, 4531

Solution: All the given numbers are 4-digit numbers so, on comparing their thousands place we get,

$5 > 4 > 3$

But thousands place of 5431 and 5231 are same. So, on comparing their hundreds place we get,

$4 > 2$

$\Rightarrow 5431 > 5231$

Hence, $5431 > 5231 > 4531 > 3451$

$\therefore$ Decreasing order is 5431, 5231, 4531, 3451.

Even and Odd Number

Even numbers

In an even number, the digits in the ones place is 0, 2, 4, 6 or 8.

Odd numbers

In an odd number, the digits in the ones place is 1, 3, 5, 7 or 9.

Expanded Form of Numbers

Example: Write the expanded form of 99999.

Solution:

99999 = 9 ten thousands + 9 thousands + 9 hundreds + 9 tens + 9 ones

$= 9 \times 10000 + 9 \times 1000 + 9 \times 100 + 9 \times 10 + 9 \times 1$

$= 90000 + 9000 + 900 + 90 + 9$

Forming Numbers

(i) To form the greatest 5-digit or 6-digit number using all the digits, arrange the digits in decreasing order.

(ii) To form the smallest 5-digit or 6-digit number using all the digits, arrange the digits in increasing order.

Example: Write the greatest and smallest 5-digit numbers using the digits 7, 2, 3, 5, 9.

Solution: Greatest number = 97532

Smallest number = 23579

Rounding Numbers

Rounding off to the nearest 10.

To round off a number to the nearest 10, we round the given number to the closest multiple of 10.

Rounding off to the nearest 100.

To round off a number to the nearest hundred, we round the given number to the closest multiple of 100.

Rounding off to the nearest 1000.

To round off a number to the nearest 1000, we round the given number to the closest multiple of 1000.

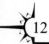

Multiple Choice Questions

1. 99,999 is the greatest _____ digit number.
   (a) 5   (b) 4
   (c) 3   (d) 2

2. Place value of 5 in 5,43,621 is _____.
   (a) 500000   (b) 5000
   (c) 50   (d) 5

3. Smallest 6-digit number is _____.
   (a) 10,0001   (b) 1,00,000
   (c) 9,99,999   (d) 99,999

4. 300000 + 20000 + 4000 + 200 + 2 = _____
   (a) 3,24,202   (b) 3,42,222
   (c) 2,34,222   (d) 3,22,432

5. Ones period includes.
   (a) Hundreds
   (b) Thousands
   (c) Ten thousands
   (d) Lakhs

6. The difference between the place values of '9' and '3' in 43549 is _____.
   (a) 2991   (b) 291
   (c) 2990   (d) 29900

7. Smallest six-digit number having 2 at hundred's place is _____.
   (a) 321201   (b) 301761
   (c) 331201   (d) 300111

8. Pick the odd one out.
   (a) Hundreds   (b) Tens
   (c) Ones   (d) Lakhs

9. We use _____ to separate the periods.
   (a) Comma   (b) Full stop
   (c) Brackets   (d) Hyphen

10. 4,37,283 is a _____ number.
    (a) 4-digit   (b) 5-digit
    (c) 6-digit   (d) 7-digit

11. The descending order of 12432, 12342, 12234, 12324 is _____.
    (a) 12324, 12432, 13342, 12234
    (b) 12432, 12342, 12324, 12234
    (c) 12234, 12324, 12342, 12432
    (d) 12432, 12324, 12342, 12234

12. Ten lakhs comes in _____ period.
    (a) Thousands   (b) Lakhs
    (c) Ones   (d) Hundreds

13. Pick odd one out.
    (a) 6, 34, 231   (b) 1, 34, 345
    (c) 1, 34, 655   (d) 23,456

14. 1 hundred thousands = _____
    (a) 1 Lakh   (b) 10 Lakh
    (c) 100 Lakh   (d) 1000 Lakh

15. Ninety-two thousands three hundred forty-five is same as _____.
    (a) 92, 435   (b) 90, 453
    (c) 92, 145   (d) 92, 345

16. 3,44,567 has _____ lakhs.
    (a) 3   (b) 4
    (c) 5   (d) 6

17. What is the estimated value of 735 nearest to 100?
    (a) 730   (b) 700
    (c) 800   (d) 750

18. What is the expanded form of 39,524?
    (a) 30000 + 9000 + 500 + 20 + 4
    (b) 3000 + 900 + 500 + 20 + 4
    (c) 30000 + 9000 + 500 + 20
    (d) 30000 + 9000 + 20 + 4

19. If 3256 is rounded off to the nearest _____, the answer will be 3000.
    (a) Tens   (b) Thousands
    (c) Hundreds   (d) None of these

20. Difference between smallest 5-digit number and smallest 4-digit number is _____.

(a) 90000   (b) 1000

(c) 9000   (d) 10000

21. The price of a car is 411140. What is the rounded off price of the car to the nearest 100?

(a) 411130   (b) 411100

(c) 411200   (d) 411150

22. The costs of three computers are ₹ 25,351, ₹ 25,400, and ₹ 30,251. What is the least cost of the computer?

(a) ₹ 29,451   (b) ₹ 25,400

(c) ₹ 30,251   (d) ₹ 25,351

23. Ravi has got five thousand nine hundreds rupees in a lottery. What is the figure value of this amount?

(a) 590   (b) 5900

(c) 5090   (d) 5009

24. A city has a population of 894710. Rounded off the population 894710 to the nearest 1000 is.

(a) 894000   (b) 894700

(c) 895000   (d) 894600

25. Sneha has 4 slips containing these four numbers.

93543   72411   23456   43517

She wants to know which one out of these numbers contains 4 at tens place. Help her to find it.

(a) 72411   (b) 93543

(c) 43517   (d) 23456

☺ ☺ ☺

Roman numbers are used widely in our daily life. The most important and common example is watches and clocks with Roman numbers on it. Roman numerals are used to number different volumes of a book, classroom in a school and questions in a question paper or exercise.

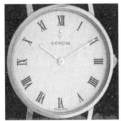

Roman Symbols

There are seven symbols used in this system which are as follows:

I, V, X, L, C, D and M

Value of the Roman symbols

Each symbol has a corresponding value:

Roman Symbol		
I	stands for	1
V	stands for	5
X	stands for	10
L	stands for	50
C	stands for	100
D	stands for	500
M	stands for	1000

Note: There is no symbol for zero in the Roman numeral system.

Rules to form Roman Numerals

1. When certain Roman numerals are repeated, the value of the resulting numeral is equal to their sum.

   III = 1 + 1 + 1 = 3

   XX = 10 + 10 = 20

2. Roman numerals read from left to right, larger values to the left and work to the smaller values on the right.

3. If a lesser numeral is before a greater number, the lesser is always subtracted from the greater numeral. For example,

   IV = 5 – 1 = 4

4. If a lesser numeral is after a greater numeral, the two numerals are added. For example, VI = 5 + 1 = 6

5. I and V can only modify up to X. For example, 49 is not written as IL, rather you first write 40 as XL and then write 9 as IX. Put them together as 49 = 40 + 9 = XLIX.

6. X and L can only modify up to C. For example, 490 is not written as XD. First you write 400 as CD and then you write 90 as XC. Put them together as

   490 = 400 + 90 = CDXC.

7. C and D can only modify up to M. For example, 950 is not written as LM, rather

you first write 900 as CM and then add L for 50. So, 950 = CML.

Note:

(i) V, L and D can not be repeated.

(ii) No roman numeral can come together more than three times. It is wrong to write IIII = 4.

(iii) The symbol V can never be written on the left of any greater value symbol.

Shortcuts to Problem Solving

1. An accurate way to write the Roman numbers is to first take the thousands, hundreds, tens and ones.

   For example, to write 1999 in Roman numeral, first write one thousand as M, nine hundred as CM, ninety as XC, nine as IX. Combine all these: MCMXCIX

2. Develop a mnemonic device to remember the order of Roman numerals.

   Think 'MeDiCaLXaVIer'. It has the Roman numerals in order from 1000 to 1.

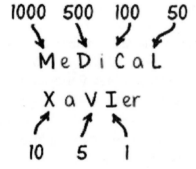

Another common mnemonic like 'I Value Xylo-phones Like Cows Dig Milk' puts the Roman numerals I, V, X, L, C, D and M in order from smallest to largest. If you have problem only in remembering larger numbers, it may help you to remember that 'C' is equivalent to 'century' and 'M' is equivalent to 'millennium': 100 and 1000, respectively.

3. Write the six pairs of subtractive Roman numeral on a notecard along with their equivalents in Roman numerals, 'IV' is equal to 4, 'IX' is equal to 9, 'XL' is equal to 40, 'XC' is equal to 90, 'CD' is equal to 400 and 'CM' is equal to 900. These are called 'subtractive' because the first letter is "subtracted" from the second. Keep the notecard visible at all times so you know to recognize these pairs when they appear.

Example: Shraddha wants to convert her friend's year of birth (1989) into roman numbers. Can you help her to do so?

Solution: Break 1989 into 1000, 900, 80 and 9, then do each conversion.

1000 = M	900 = CM
80 = LXXX	9 = IX

So, 1989 = 1000 + 900 + 80 + 9 = MCMLXXXIX

Multiple Choice Questions

1. Romans used the numbers for trading and _____.
   (a) Commerce
   (b) Finance
   (c) Law
   (d) Exporting

2. Addition is only applicable when the first symbol is _____ than the second, third.
   (a) Greater
   (b) Smaller
   (c) Equal
   (d) Greater than equal to

3. **Statement A:** When the principle of addition is used, a symbol can be used only three times.
   Statement B: When the principle of addition is used, a symbol can be used only 1 time.
   (a) A is correct
   (b) B is correct
   (c) Both are correct
   (d) Both are incorrect

4. Pick the odd one out.
   V, IV, X, XI, VIIII.
   (a) IV   (b) XI
   (c) V   (d) VIIII

5. Pick the odd one out.
   I, V, X, L, C, D, N.
   (a) X   (b) I
   (c) C   (d) N

6. Roman numbers don't have symbol for _____.
   (a) Zero   (b) One
   (c) Two   (d) Three

7. When a symbol appears after larger symbol, it is _____
   (a) Added
   (b) Subtracted
   (c) Multiplied
   (d) Divided

8. Subtraction is only applicable when the first symbol is _____ than the second one.
   (a) Less
   (b) More
   (c) Equal to
   (d) Less than equal to

9. Convert CVI into numbers.
   (a) 100   (b) 105
   (c) 106   (d) 110

10. Convert 1400 into numbers.
    (a) MCD   (b) MC
    (c) MD   (d) M

11. Convert MXVI into numbers.
    (a) 1016   (b) 101
    (c) 1006   (d) 1000

12. Pick the odd one out.
    C, XL, LXXXX
    (a) C
    (b) XL
    (c) LXXXX
    (d) None of these

13. MMLXIII – CDLXXXVI is equal to.
    (a) MDLXXVII
    (b) MDLXXVI
    (c) MDLXV
    (d) MDLXVIII

14. DCCCLIX + XXVII + DCCCXLII =?
    (a) MDCCXXVI
    (b) MDCCXXVIII
    (c) MDCXXVII
    (d) MDCCXXVII

15. Write 830 as a roman numeral.
    (a) DCCCXX
    (b) DCXXX
    (c) DCCCXXX
    (d) DCCXXX

16. Write 2990 as a roman numeral.
    (a) MMCXC   (b) MCMXC
    (c) MMCMXC   (d) MMCMC

17. Convert the statement into Roman numbers
    5 × 4
    (a) V × IV = XX
    (b) V × IV= VIV
    (c) V × IIII = XX
    (d) V × IV = VVVV

18. Solve DVI – XXIV = ?
    (a) CDLXXXI   (b) CDLXXXII
    (c) CDLXXII   (d) CDLXXX

19. Observe the pattern of given numbers

    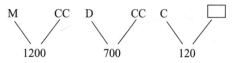

    Which Roman numeral must fill the blank box?
    (a) IV   (b) X
    (c) XL   (d) XX

20. Identify the greatest Roman number.
    660 (a) DCLX   (b) CDXL 660
    (c) DCXL   (d) CDCX

21. Four students Pandu, Kittu, Sweety and Chintu wrote Roman numerals on their slates as shown.

    32 XXXII XXXIX XXV XVIII
       Pandu Kittu Sweety Chintu
    Who wrote the least number?
    (a) Pandu   (b) Kittu
    (c) Sweety   (d) Chintu

22. Titu had M grapes. He gave CD grapes to Meena. How many grapes does Titu have ?
    (a) DC   (b) D
    (c) C   (d) DCC

23. Sumit has VIII roses. Aman has VII more roses than Sumit. How many roses does Aman have?
    (a) XII   (b) XV
    (c) IVX   (d) XVI

24. Pooja has VI Barbie dolls. She has V dresses for each doll. How many Barbie dresses does she have together?
    (a) XXX   (b) XXV
    (c) XXIX   (d) XXXV

25. Himanshu had XV balls. He gave V balls to his friend. How many balls does Himanshu have now?
    (a) IX   (b) XI
    (c) X   (d) VIII

☺ ☺ ☺

Addition

Learning Objectives:

In this chapter, students will learn about:

- Properties of addition
- Addition (Without Regrouping)
- Addition (With Regrouping)
- Estimating the sum

Addition

Combining two or more objects of same kind is known as addition.

Terminology

Addend: The numbers that are to be added are called addends.

Sum: The result obtained after addition is called sum.

ADDEND + ADDEND = SUM

For example, 4550 + 1120 = 5670

Here,

4550 = Addend

1120 = Addend

5670 = Sum

Properties of Addition

(i) When we add 1 to any number, the sum is always its successor.

For example,

9,74,357 + 1 = 9,74,358 where 9,74,358 is the successor of 9,74,357

(ii) When we add 0 to a number, the sum is the number itself.

For example, 29,937 + 0 = 29,937

(iii) If we change the order of numbers while adding, the sum does not change.

For example,

70,321 + 60,230 = 1,30,5551

Also, 60,230 + 70,321 = 1,30,551

Thus, 70,321 + 60,230 = 60,230 + 70,321

Example: Prove 25,000 + 34,000 is same as 34,000 + 25,000

Solution: Addend 1 = 25,000

Addend 2 = 34,000

Sum = 59,000

If we interchange the addends with each other that is 34,000 becomes addend 1 and 25,000 becomes addend 2. The sum remains the same.

That is, 34,000 + 25,000 = 59,000

Hence, we can say that if the order of the numbers to be added is changed, the sum will remain the same.

(iv) When three or more numbers are added the sum of remains the same regardless of the way addends are grouped.

For example,

(90,000 + 60,000) + 50,000

= 1,50,000 + 50,000 = 2,00,000

Also, 90,000 + (60,000 + 50,000)

= 90,000 + 1,00,000 = 2,00,000

Thus, (90,000 + 60,000) + 50,000

= 90,000 + (60,000 + 50,000)

Note: The sum is always greater than the numbers being added, except when one of the number's being added is zero.

Addition (Without Regrouping)

Shraddha went to the zoo, she found that there were 92163 animals and 10822 birds.

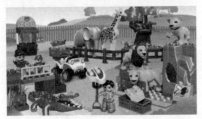

She wants to know, what is the total number of animals and birds in the zoo. Let us help her to do so.

Number of animals in the zoo = 92163

Number of birds in the zoo = 10822

Total number of animals and birds in the zoo = 92163 + 10822

We can also write this in place value columns as follows:

TTh	Th	H	T	O
9	2	1	6	3
+ 1	0	8	2	2

Step 1. Start with ones column and proceed towards the left.

Adding 3 and 2 on ones column gives 5 as shown below:

TTh	Th	H	T	O
9	2	1	6	3
+ 1	0	8	2	2
				5

Step 2. Now moving to the tens column, 6 + 2 = 8

TTh	Th	H	T	O
9	2	1	6	3
+ 1	0	8	2	2
			8	5

Step 3. In the Hundred column, 1 + 8 = 9

TTh	Th	H	T	O
9	2	1	6	3
+ 1	0	8	2	2
		9	8	5

Step 4. In the thousands column, 2 + 0 = 2

TTh	Th	H	T	O
9	2	1	6	3
+ 1	0	8	2	2
	2	9	8	5

Step 5. Lastly, in the ten thousands column, 9 + 1 = 10

TTh	Th	H	T	O
9	2	1	6	3
+ 1	0	8	2	2
10	2	9	8	5

Hence, total number of animals and birds in the zoo is 102985.

This kind of addition is known as addition without regrouping. Now we will learn how to do addition with regrouping.

Addition (With Regrouping)

In a month, 87125 men and 53799 women went to the beach. We will find out the total number of people who visited the beach.

Number of men = 87125

Number of women = 53799

Total number of people = 87125 + 53799

Let us write this in place value column as follows:

TTh	Th	H	T	O
8	7	1	2	5
+ 5	3	7	9	9

Step 1. Adding the digits on ones column, $5 + 9 = 14$

We will write 4 in the ones column and 1 will be regrouped to tens column as shown below:

TTh	Th	H	T	O
			1	
8	7	1	2	5
+ 5	3	7	9	9
				4

Step 2. In the tens column, $1 + 2 + 9 = 12$

Again 1 will be regrouped to hundreds column as shown below:

TTh	Th	H	T	O
			1	
8	7	1	2	5
+ 5	3	7	9	9
			2	4

Step 3. In the hundreds column, $1 + 1 + 7 = 9$

TTh	Th	H	T	O
		1	1	
8	7	1	2	5
+ 5	3	7	9	9
		9	2	4

Step 4. Moving to the thousands column, $7 + 3 = 10$

TTh	Th	H	T	O
		1	1	
8	7	1	2	5
+ 5	3	7	9	9
	0	9	2	4

Step 5. Lastly, in the ten thousands column, $1 + 8 + 5 = 14$.

TTh	Th	H	T	O
1		1	1	
8	7	1	2	5
+ 5	3	7	9	9
14	0	9	2	4

Therefore, total number of people is 140924

This form of addition is known as addition with regrouping.

Estimating the sum

By estimating the sum, we get an approximate sum of the given numbers.

To calculate the estimated sum, find the sum of the rounded off volume of each of the addends.

Example: Find the estimated sum of 72,321 and 53,461 by rounding off to nearest 100

Solution: 72,321 rounded off to the nearest 100 is 72,300.

53,461 rounded off to the nearest 100 is 53,500

$72,300 + 53,500 = 1,25,800$

Thus, the estimated sum of 72,321 and 53,461 is 1,25,800

Amazing Addition Patterns

A. **Sum of three consecutive numbers differ by 3.**

$1 + 2 + 3 = 6$
$2 + 3 + 4 = 9$
$3 + 4 + 5 = 12$
$4 + 5 + 6 = 15$

B. **Sum of five consecutive numbers differ by 5.**

$1 + 2 + 3 + 4 + 5 = 15$
$2 + 3 + 4 + 5 + 6 = 20$
$3 + 4 + 5 + 6 + 7 = 25$

C. $1 + 2 + 3 + 4 + 5 + 6 + 7 + 8 + 9 + 10 = 55$

Sum of 1 to 10 = 55

Sum of 11 to 20 = 155

Sum of 21 to 30 = 255

Sum of 31 to 40 = 355

Trick

Aim for ten. If you see any number close to ten, then break the other number so that you reach ten.

Example: $8 + 5 = ?$

8 is 2 away from 10, so $8 + 2 = 10$

Now 5 becomes 3.

Therefore, $10 + 3 = 13$

Multiple Choice Questions

1. The sum is always _____ than the numbers being added, except of the numbers being added is _____.
   - (a) Greater, zero
   - (b) Less, zero
   - (c) Greater, one
   - (d) Less, one

2. If we change the order of the numbers being added, the _____ does not change.
   - (a) Sum
   - (b) Difference
   - (c) Multiplication
   - (d) Division

3. $0 + 33456 =$ _____
   - (a) 0
   - (b) 33456
   - (c) 34346
   - (d) 30456

4. If we add _____ to any number, the sum remains the same.
   - (a) Zero
   - (b) One
   - (c) Two
   - (d) Three

5. If we add _____ to any number, the sum is always its successor.
   - (a) Zero
   - (b) One
   - (c) Two
   - (d) Three

6. $4325 + 1 =$ _____
   - (a) 4325
   - (b) 4326
   - (c) 4327
   - (d) 4328

7. Addend + _____ = _____
   - (a) Addend, Sum
   - (b) Minuend, Sum
   - (c) Subtrahend, Sum
   - (d) Difference, Sum

8. Pick the odd one out.
   - (a) Sum
   - (b) Plus
   - (c) Increase
   - (d) Difference

9. On adding two numbers, the result obtained is called _____.
   - (a) Sum
   - (b) difference
   - (c) addend
   - (d) minuend

10. The numbers to be added are known as _____.
    - (a) sum
    - (b) difference
    - (c) addend
    - (d) minuend

11. If 🍎 + 🍎 + 🍎 + 🍎 + 🍎 = 50 oranges and 🍎 + 🍎 + 🍎 + 🍎 = 160 fruits, then 🍎 stands for _____ fruits.
    - (a) 30
    - (b) 40
    - (c) 50
    - (d) 20

12. What is the estimated sum of 43,535, 50,723 and 73,758 by rounding off the numbers to the nearest 10 ?
    - (a) 168020
    - (b) 168030
    - (c) 158020
    - (d) 178040

13. Sum of $32,145 + 2000$ is _____.
    - (a) 34,145
    - (b) 34,140
    - (c) 34,150
    - (d) 34,160

14. $2,40,532 + 93,777 = 93,777 +$ _____
    - (a) 2,40,532
    - (b) 93,777
    - (c) 2,41,531
    - (d) 92,761

15. $(45,773 + 73,921) + 53,773 =$ _____ $+$ $(73,921 + 53,773)$
    - (a) 53,773
    - (b) 45,772
    - (c) 73,921
    - (d) 45,773

16. Pick the odd one out.
    - (a) Addend
    - (b) Sum
    - (c) Total
    - (d) Difference

17. $516 +$ _____ $= 516$
    - (a) 0
    - (b) 1
    - (c) 2
    - (d) 516

18. $1005 + \underline{\quad} = 1006$
    - (a) 0
    - (b) 1
    - (c) 2
    - (d) 1005

19. Identify the addends and the sum.
    $5674 + 6 = 5680$
    - (a) Addends = 5674, 5680, Sum = 6
    - (b) Addends = 5680, 6, Sum = 5674
    - (c) Addends = 5674, 6, Sum = 5680
    - (d) Addends = 5674, Sum = 5680

20. $45,001 + 93,777 = \underline{\quad}$
    - (a) 1,38,770
    - (b) 1,28,778
    - (c) 1,38,778
    - (d) 1,38,678

21. The annual fees of Shubhra is ₹ 5372 and the annual fees of Shraddha is ₹ 4352. What is their total fees altogether?
    - (a) ₹ 9734
    - (b) ₹ 9724
    - (c) ₹ 9624
    - (d) ₹ 9825

22. A car travelled from town A to B and then from town B to C. The distance between towns A and B is 4364 km and between B and C is 5473 km. What is the total distance travelled by car?
    - (a) 9834 km
    - (b) 6453 km
    - (c) 9837 km
    - (d) 5463 km

23. Swati purchased a dress for ₹ 5473 and a pair of footwear of ₹ 2335. What is the total amount she spent?
    - (a) ₹ 8708
    - (b) ₹ 7808
    - (c) ₹ 7800
    - (d) ₹ 7353

24. Sahil bough a chair for ₹ 12,530 and a table for ₹ 23,450. Find the rounded off sum of table and chair nearest to 100.
    - (a) ₹ 45,000
    - (b) ₹ 55,000
    - (c) ₹ 35,000
    - (d) ₹ 65,000

25. 23,567 people enrolled for dance classes in 2016 and 45,732 more people enrolled for the dance classes in 2017. How many people in all enrolled for the dance classes in both the years?
    - (a) 69209
    - (b) 60000
    - (c) 60200
    - (d) 69299

Subtraction

Learning Objectives:

In this chapter, students will learn about:

- Properties of Subtraction
- Subtraction (Without Regrouping)
- Subtraction (With Regrouping)
- Estimation of difference

Subtraction

Subtraction is taking away some objects from a given collection.

Terminology
• Minuend: The number that is to be subtracted from is called minuend.
• Subtrahend: The number that is to be subtracted is called subtrahend.
• Difference: The result obtained after subtraction is called difference.
MINUEND – SUBTRAHEND = DIFFERENCE
For example,
If 1050 – 1020 = 30
Minuend = 1050
Subtrahend = 1020
Difference = 30

Properties of Subtraction

(i) When we subtract a number from itself, the difference is always zero.

For example, $76884 - 76884 = 0$

(ii) When we subtract zero from a number, the difference is the number itself.

(iii) If 1 is subtracted from a number, the difference is the predecessor of the given number.

For example, $51,933 - 1 = 51,932$

Uses of Subtraction

(i) To find out how many are left.

Example: In a singing competition, 25,321 students out of 75,000 qualified for the next round. How many students were left unselected?

Solution: We have to find the number of students who were left unselected. Whenever we have to find how many are left we use subtraction.

Therefore, the number of students left unselected = Total number of students – Number of students selected

$= 75,000 - 25,321 = 49,679$

(ii) To compare groups.

Example: There are 7,21,000 apartments in the town A and 9,00,500 apartments in the town B. How many more apartments are there in the town B than town A?

Solution: We have two groups:

(a) Town A   (b) Town B

Now to compare the apartments of two groups, we will subtract the smaller group from the larger group.

This is shown as follows:

$$9,00,500$$
$$-7,21,000$$
$$1,79,5000$$

Thus, 1,79,500 more apartments are there in town B than in town A.

(iii) To find what does not belong to a group.

Example: A farmer loaded a truck with 51,129 onions. On the way, some onions fell on the road. On unloading, the farmer found that there are only 10,000 onions. Find out how many onions fell from the truck.

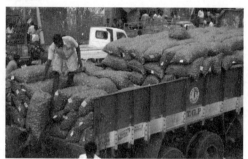

Solution: Here we know the original number and the number which is left over. We need to find the number of onions that fell from the truck.

This can be written as follows:

Therefore, the number of onions which fell from the truck are:

$$51,129 - 10,000 = 41,129$$

(iv) To find out how many are needed.

Example: A thirsty crow needs 31,255 pebbles to put in the pot to raise the water level. But he has only 255 pebbles. How many more pebbles does he need?

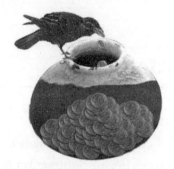

Solution: $225 + ? = 31255$

The number of pebbles required by crow to raise the water level is:

$$31255 - 255 = 31000$$

Subtraction (Without Regrouping)

Example: There are 12549 seats in a circus tent. 2138 people came to see the circus show. How many seats were left vacant?

Solution: To find out the number of vacant seats we will use subtraction as follows:

No. of vacant seats = Total no. of seats − no. of seats occupied by people = 12549 − 2138

TTh	Th	H	T	O
1	2	5	4	9
−	2	1	3	8
1	0	4	1	1

Therefore, 10411 seats were left vacant.

Subtraction (With Regrouping)

Example: Out of 21380, 1619 people who came to see the circus, were adults. Remaining were childeren. Find out how many children were there ?

Solution: Total number of children = Total number of people − Total number of adults
= 21380 − 1619

This can also be written as:

TTh	Th	H	T	O
1	0	13	7	10
2	1	3	3	0
–		1	6	1	9
1	9	7	6	1

Note: We can check subtraction using addition. If the sum of the subtrahend and the difference gives the minuend, then the subtraction is done correctly.

Example: Find the difference and check your answer for the following:

TTh	Th	H	T	O
7	9	3	2	1
– 5	6	0	1	3

Solution:

TTh	Th	H	T	O
7	9	3	2	1
– 5	6	0	1	3
2	3	3	0	8

Checking the answer:

TTh	Th	H	T	O
2	3	3	0	8
+ 5	6	0	1	3
7	9	3	2	1

Thus, answer is correct.

Estimating the difference

By estimating the difference, we get an approximate difference of the given numbers.

To calculate the estimated difference, find the difference of the rounded off value of the minuend and the subtrahend.

Example: Solve $40{,}537 - 11{,}200 + 77{,}939$.

Solution: Subtracting 11,200 from 40,537.

4	0	5	3	7
– 1	1	2	0	0
2	9	3	3	7

Now, adding 29,337 and 77,939.

2	9	3	3	7
+ 7	7	9	3	9
10	7	2	7	6

Thus, $40{,}537 - 11{,}200 + 77{,}939 = 107276$

Multiple Choice Questions

1. _____ is taking away some objects from a given collection.
   - (a) Addition
   - (b) Subtraction
   - (c) Multiplication
   - (d) Division

2. The result obtained after subtraction is called _____.
   - (a) Minuend
   - (b) Subtrahend
   - (c) Difference
   - (d) Sum

3. _____ is the number that is to be subtracted from.
   - (a) Minuend
   - (b) Subtrahend
   - (c) Difference
   - (d) Sum

4. Pick the odd one out.
   - (a) Minus
   - (b) Less
   - (c) Difference
   - (d) Sum

5. Find the difference of 5,62,562 – 23,425.
   - (a) 539137
   - (b) 539136
   - (c) 530127
   - (d) 439136

6. When we subtract a number from itself, the difference is always _____.
   - (a) Zero
   - (b) One
   - (c) Two
   - (d) Itself

7. Subtract 3,20,316 from the sum of 4,30,408 and 93,415.
   - (a) 2,04,506
   - (b) 7,05,601
   - (c) 2,03,507
   - (d) 7,05,701

8. When we subtract _____ from a number, the difference is the number itself.
   - (a) Zero
   - (b) One
   - (c) Two
   - (d) Itself

9. If $\square + \square + \square + \square = 2400$ and $1000 - \square = \bigcirc$, then the value of $\bigcirc$ is _____.
   - (a) 400
   - (b) 600
   - (c) 1000
   - (d) 200

10. Read the statements carefully and choose the correct option.

    Statement A: Minuend – Subtrahend = Difference

    Statement B: Minuend – Difference = Subtrahend
    - (a) Statement A is true b is false.
    - (b) Statement B is true A is false.
    - (c) Both the statements are true.
    - (d) Both the statements are false.

11. Find the subtrahend:
    $1000 - ? = 900$
    - (a) 10
    - (b) 0
    - (c) 90
    - (d) 1

12. Tick the correct option.
    - i. $999 - 0 = 999$
    - ii. $999 - 999 = 0$
    - (a) i is correct.
    - (b) ii is correct.
    - (c) Both are correct.
    - (d) Both are incorrect.

13. Estimate the difference between 32,532 and 12,200 by rounding off the given numbers to the nearest 1000.
    - (a) 11000
    - (b) 21000
    - (c) 10000
    - (d) 5000

14. Tick the correct option.
    - i. Subtraction is used to find out how many are left.
    - ii. Subtraction is used to find out the total amount.
    - (a) i is correct.
    - (b) ii is correct.
    - (c) Both are correct.
    - (d) Both are incorrect.

15. Solve the problem.

    $11015 + ? = 11025$

    (a) 10   (b) 15

    (c) 25   (d) 5

16. We use subtraction when we have to find how many more to be _____ to get the given number.

    (a) Added

    (b) Subtracted

    (c) Multiplied

    (d) Divided

17. Estimate the following to the nearest 10.

    $53,332 - 43,325$

    (a) 10000   (b) 1000

    (c) 100   (d) 100000

18. Solve using shortcut.

    $8000 - 1584$

    (a) 6416   (b) 6400

    (c) 1584   (d) 6410

19. _____ $- 1 = 4,25,693$

    (a) 4,25,693   (b) 4,25,692

    (c) 4,25,694   (d) 4,25,690

20. Subtract: $9000 - 1999$

    (a) 7000   (b) 7001

    (c) 7002   (d) 7003

21. There are 34,254 red and yellow roses. 13,245 roses are yellow in colour. Estimate the number of red roses to the nearest 100.

    (a) 21100   (b) 2100

    (c) 211100   (d) 21101

22. Shraddha has a book of 119 pages. She has read 59 pages. How many pages are left to be read?

    (a) 60   (b) 59

    (c) 119   (d) 58

23. A poultry farm sends 1647 eggs to the market in a van. On the way 234 eggs broke. How many eggs were left in the van?

    (a) 1413   (b) 1234

    (c) 1647   (d) 234

24. Talwar family consumes 1000 kgs wheat in a year whereas, Mehra family consumes 959 kgs of wheat in a year. How much more kgs of wheat does Talwar family consume?

    (a) 41   (b) 45

    (c) 40   (d) 39

25. In the parking area, there were 2198 cars and 1212 bikes. How many more cars were there than bikes?

    (a) 986   (b) 987

    (c) 988   (d) 989

☺ ☺ ☺

Multiplication

> **Learning Objectives:**
> In this chapter, students will learn about:
> * Properties of Multiplication
> * Multiplication (Traditional Method)
> * Multiplication by 10, 20, 100 and 1000
> * Multiplication by 20, 30, 40...
> * Estimation of the Product

Multiplication

Multiplication is used in daily household activities. For example, if 2 glasses of water is required to cook 1 glass of rice, then how many glasses of water are required to cook 5 glasses of rice? Another example is, 72 people can sit in one train compartment. How many people can sit on the train with 15 such compartments? These queries are well answered by multiplication computing.

Multiplication is the process of finding the product of any two numbers. It is a mathematical operation that indicates how many times a number is added to itself.

Terminology
* **Multiplicand:** The number to be multiplied is called the multiplicand.
* **Multiplier:** The number by which we multiply is called the multiplier.
* **Product:** The result after multiplication is known as the product.

Properties of Multiplication
(i) Zero Property

When we multiply any number by 0, the product is always 0.

For example, $356 \times 0 = 0$

(ii) Property of 1

When we multiply any number by 1, the product is the number itself.

For example, $255 \times 1 = 255$

(iii) Order Property

The product of two numbers grouped in any order remains the same.

For example, $943 \times 11 = 11 \times 943 = 10,373$

(iv) The product of three numbers grouped in any order remains the same.

$92 \times 14 \times 5 = (92 \times 14) \times 5$
$= 92 \times (14 \times 5) = 6,440$

Multiplication (Traditional Method)

We will multiply 56 and 551. We could simply keep adding 551s together until we have 56 lots of 551, but that could take a very long time. Instead, we use the following method:

Step 1: Set the multiplication out as follows.

H	T	O
5	5	1
×	5	6

Note: that the number with the less number of digits goes at the bottom.

Step 2: Multiply 551 by 6.

	H	T	O
	5	5	1
×		5	6
3	**3**	**0**	**6**

The result of 6 × 551 is shown in bold.

Step 3: Next, multiply 551 by 50. This is the same as multiplying 551 by 5 and by 10. We place a zero to the right and then write down the result of 5 × 551.

	5	5	1
×		5	6
3	3	0	6
2	**7**	**5**	**5**	**0**

The result of 5 × 551 is shown in bold and the additional zero has been also shown in bold.

Step 4: Finally, add these two rows together to give the final product.

		5	5	1
	×		5	6
	3	3	0	6
2	7	5	5	0
3	0	8	5	6

The final product for 56 × 551 is 30856.

Similarly, we can multiply a 3-digit number by a 3-digit number.

Example: Multiply 430 by 111.

Solution:

		4	3	0
	×	1	1	1
		4	3	0
	4	3	0	×
+	4	3	0	×	×
	4	7	7	3	0

We can also multiply a 4-digit number by a 1-digit number or by a 2-digit number.

Example: Multiply 2016 by 3.
Solution:

	2	0	1	6
		×		3
	6	0	4	8

Long multiplication or Box method

Multiplying 56 × 551 by using the box method. This method begins by splitting each of the numbers:

551 = 500 + 50 + 1
56 = 50 + 6

Next step is forming grid. Like this:

	500	50	1
50			
6			

Now multiply a number from the top edge with a number from the left edge and place the product in the appropriate cell in the table.

For example, 50 × 500 = 25000

In the following steps continue filling the values in similar way and you will get something like this:

	500	50	1
50	25000	2500	50
6	3000	300	6

Lastly, add together all the numbers in the grid to get the final product.

56 × 551 = 25000 + 2500 + 50 + 3000 + 300 + 6 = 30856

Therefore, 56 × 551 = 30856

Multiplication by 10, 100 and 1000

When we multiply given numbers by 10, 100, 1000 and so on (powers of ten), we can simply write as many zeros on the product as there are in the factor 10, 100, 1000, etc.

For example, 2 × 10 = 20, 51 × 100 = 5100, 322 × 100 = 32200

Multiplication by 20, 30, 40....

To multiply a given number by 20, 30, 40, ... we multiply the number by 2, 3, 4, ... and then we put one zero to the right of the product and get the product.

For example,

$15 \times 20 = 15 \times 2$ tens $= (15 \times 2)$ tens $= 30$ tens $= 300$

Some Interesting Patterns

(i) $37 \times 3 \times 1 = 111$

     $37 \times 3 \times 2 = 222$

     $37 \times 3 \times 3 = 333$ and so on

(ii) $15873 \times 7 \times 1 = 111111$

     $15873 \times 7 \times 2 = 222222$

     $15873 \times 7 \times 3 = 333333$ and so on

(iii) $9 \times 0 + 1 = 1$

     $9 \times 1 + 2 = 11$

     $9 \times 2 + 3 = 21$

     $9 \times 3 + 4 = 31$

     $9 \times 4 + 5 = 41$ and so on

Estimating the product

By estimating a product, we get an approximate value of the product.

To estimate a product, round off each number to the nearest 10 or 1000 and then find the product of the rounded values.

Multiple Choice Questions

1. Multiplicand × Multiplier = ?
   - (a) Product
   - (b) Difference
   - (c) Sum
   - (d) Addend

2. Multiplication is the short form of repeated _____
   - (a) Multiplication
   - (b) Division
   - (c) Addition
   - (d) Subtraction

3. $43243 \times 0 =$ _____
   - (a) 43432
   - (b) 0
   - (c) 44432
   - (d) 42432

4. $66 \times 1 =$ _____
   - (a) 1766
   - (b) 1767
   - (c) 1765
   - (d) 0

5. $7074 \times 21 = 21 \times$ _____
   - (a) 7074
   - (b) 2121
   - (c) 1554
   - (d) 1

6. $543 \times 10 =$ _____
   - (a) 5430
   - (b) 5400
   - (c) 543
   - (d) 54300

7. $23 \times 100 =$ _____
   - (a) 2300
   - (b) 23000
   - (c) 230
   - (d) 23

8. $365 \times$ _____ $= 74 \times 365$
   - (a) 65
   - (b) 74
   - (c) 0
   - (d) 10

9. $11 \times 11 =$ _____
   - (a) 111
   - (b) 121
   - (c) 131
   - (d) 141

10. $25 \times 25 =$ _____
    - (a) 325
    - (b) 425
    - (c) 525
    - (d) 625

11. Pick the odd one out: 5, 10, 15, 20, 24
    - (a) 5
    - (b) 15
    - (c) 20
    - (d) 24

12. Pick the odd one out: 11, 22, 32, 44, 55
    - (a) 11
    - (b) 22
    - (c) 32
    - (d) 44

13. $22 \times 5 =$ _____
    - (a) 100
    - (b) 105
    - (c) 110
    - (d) 115

14. _____ $\times 5 = 50$
    - (a) 5
    - (b) 10
    - (c) 15
    - (d) 20

15. $9 \times 400 =$ _____
    - (a) 36
    - (b) 360
    - (c) 3600
    - (d) 36000

16. $9 \times 9 =$ _____
    - (a) 9
    - (b) 18
    - (c) 81
    - (d) 99

17. Estimate the product of 693 and 312 by rounding off the numbers to the nearest 100.
    - (a) 210000
    - (b) 180000
    - (c) 240000
    - (d) 150000

18. $966 \times 20 =$ _____.
    - (a) 19320
    - (b) 1932
    - (c) 1930
    - (d) 19300

19. $987 \times 9 =$ _____
    - (a) 8888
    - (b) 8883
    - (c) 3888
    - (d) 8833

20. $796 \times 7 =$ _____
    - (a) 5572
    - (b) 2257
    - (c) 5277
    - (d) 2527

21. There are 79 crayons in one box. How many crayons are in 93 boxes?
    - (a) 6510
    - (b) 6520
    - (c) 6530
    - (d) 6540

22. Titu, Jeeti, Janu and Lalli have 250 poke-mon cards each. How many cards do they have in all?
    (a) 1000   (b) 250
    (c) 4   (d) 1100

23. A cricket stadium has 456 rows with 200 seats in each row. How many seats are there in the stadium?
    (a) 91200   (b) 91000
    (c) 81200   (d) 90200

24. Golu bought 6 bags of jellybeans. If each bag has 24 jellybeans, what is the total amount he has?
    (a) 124 jellybeans   (b) 144 jellybeans
    (c) 114 jellybeans   (d) 140 jellybeans

25. Estimate the total number of toys by rounding off to the nearest 10 if there are 143 rows with 109 toys in each row.
    (a) 14000   (b) 1400
    (c) 140   (d) 14

Division

Learning Objectives:

In this chapter, students will learn about:

- Properties of Division
- Long Division
- Imperfect Division
- Division by 10,100 and 1000
- Estimating the guotient

Division

Division is splitting into equal parts or groups. It is the result of 'fair sharing'. When we share equally we divide. Sharing and subtracting repeatedly are two of the basic ways of dividing. We also use multiplication tables in dividing.

For example, Shraddha found 25 beautiful pearls on the seashore. She collected and brought all of them home. Now she wants to put them in jewellery boxes. She can put 5 pearls in one jewellery box.

She made 1 group of 5 pearls and put them in 1 jewellery box.

She put 5 more pearls in 2nd jewellery box.

She is left with some pearls, so she put 5 pearls in another jewellery box.

She put 5 more pearls in another jewellery box.

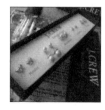 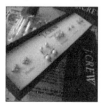 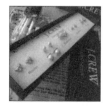 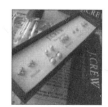

Also she put 5 more pearls in another box.

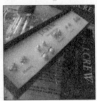 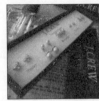 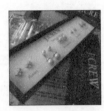 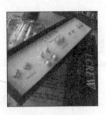

No more pearls are left. Thus, Shraddha required 5 jewellery boxes to keep the pearls. Therefore, we can say that 25 pearls into equal groups of 5 each give 5 groups.

Symbolically, we write as

$25 \div 5 = 5$

Terminology

Dividend: The number to be divided is called the dividend. It is the number you want to divide up.

Divisor: The number which divides the dividend is called the divisor.

Quotient: The result obtained after dividing one number by another is called quotient.

For example: $12 \div 6 = 2$

Here, 12 is to be divided by 6.

So, 12 is the dividend and 6 is the divisor.

On dividing 12 by 6, we get 2, which is quotient.

Properties of Division

(i)   Zero Property

If zero is divided by any number, the result is always zero.

For example, $0 \div 5 = 0$

(ii) Any number divided by zero is not defined.

(iii) Property of 1:

If any number is divided by 1, the result is the number itself.

Example: Bhola's family has gone to the market so he is alone at home. There are 9 cookies kept in the kitchen. How many cookies will Bhola get to eat?

Solution: Here, Bhola can eat all the 9 cookies as there is no one else to share the cookies.

Therefore, 9 cookies are to be divided amongst one person.

That is, $9 \div 1 = 9$

(iv) Dividing a number by itself.

If any number is divided by itself, the resull will always be 1.

Example: Bhola's family is back at home. They have brought a pizza for all of them. There are total 6 members in the family including Bhola. The pizza is divided into 6 equal parts. How many parts will each member get?

6 equal parts are to be shared amongst 6 members.

Solution: That is, $6 \div 6 = 1$

Each member will get 1 part of pizza.

Therefore, we can say that any number divided by itself gives 1 as the quotient.

Note:
- Remainder must always be smaller than the divisor.
- We can check result by following the rule:

(Quotient × Divisor) + Remainder = Dividend

Long Division

Let's see how division is done with help of an example. We will divide 425 by 25 here.

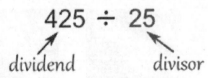

Step 1: Since 4 cannot be divided by 25, divide 42 by 25. Now $25 \times 1 = 25$

Write 1 in the quotient and 25 below 42 and then subtract.

$$
\begin{array}{r}
1 \\
25\overline{)\,425} \\
-25 \\
\hline
17
\end{array}
$$

Step 2: Bring down 5. Divide 175 by 25. Since $25 \times 7 = 175$. So, write 7 in the quotient and 175 below 175 and then subtract.

$$
\begin{array}{r}
17 \\
25\overline{)\,425} \\
-25\!\downarrow \\
\hline
175 \\
-175 \\
\hline
0
\end{array}
$$

Thus, quotient = 17 and remainder = 0.

Imperfect Division (with Remainder)

To understand this we are taking example similar to the one taken above: $435 \div 25$

Step 1: Since 4 cannot be divided by 25, divide 43 by 25. Now, $25 \times 1 = 25$

Write 1 in the quotient place and 25 below 43 and then subtract.

$$
\begin{array}{r}
1 \\
25\overline{)\,435} \\
25 \\
\hline
18
\end{array}
$$

Step 2: Bring down 5. Divide 185 by 25 Since $25 \times 7 = 175$. So, write 7 in the quotient and 175 below 185 and then subtract.

$$
\begin{array}{r}
17 \\
25\overline{)\,435} \\
-25\!\downarrow \\
\hline
185 \\
-175 \\
\hline
10
\end{array}
$$

Thus, quotient = 17 and remainder = 10

Division by 10, 100 and 1000

(i) Any number divided by 10 gives the ones digit as remainder and remaining digits as the quotient.

For example, on dividing 9224 by 10, we get, quotient = 922 and remainder = 4

(ii) If a number divided by 100, then the digits at ones and tens places together form the remainder and remaining digits form the quotient.

For example, on dividing 7624 by 100 we get, quotient = 76 and remainder = 24

(iii) Similarly, if a number is divided by 1000, then the digits at ones, tens and hundreds place together form the remainder and remaining digits form the quotient.

For example, on dividing 17432 by 1000 we get quotient = 17 and remainder = 432

Interesting Patterns in Division

As the dividend increases, the quotient also increases.

$$4 \div 2 = 2$$
$$40 \div 2 = 20$$
$$400 \div 2 = 200$$
$$4000 \div 2 = 2000$$

As the divisor decreases, the quotient also decreases.

$$4000 \div 2 = 2000$$
$$4000 \div 20 = 200$$
$$4000 \div 200 = 20$$
$$4000 \div 2000 = 2$$

Estimating the quotient

By estimating a quotient, we get an approximate value of the quotient.

To estimate a quotient, divide the rounded values of dividend and divisor.

Multiple Choice Questions

1. When we share equally, we _____.
   - (a) Add
   - (b) Subtract
   - (c) Multiply
   - (d) Divide

2. The number to be divided is called the _____.
   - (a) Quotient
   - (b) Divisor
   - (c) Dividend
   - (d) Remainder

3. After dividing a number, the leftover is called _____.
   - (a) Quotient
   - (b) Divisor
   - (c) Dividend
   - (d) Remainder

4. What is the remainder when 3527 is divided by 10 ?
   - (a) 3
   - (b) 5
   - (c) 2
   - (d) 7

5. $9000 \div 1000 =$ _____
   - (a) 90
   - (b) 1
   - (c) 10
   - (d) 9

6. $0 \div 56 =$ _____
   - (a) 0
   - (b) 1
   - (c) 56
   - (d) None of these

7. _____ is the number that we divide by.
   - (a) Dividend
   - (b) Divisor
   - (c) Quotient
   - (d) Remainder

8. $828 \div 2 = 424$. Here, 424 is the _____.
   - (a) Quotient
   - (b) Remainder
   - (c) Dividend
   - (d) Divisor

9. If any number is divided by _____, the result is the number itself.
   - (a) Zero
   - (b) One
   - (c) Two
   - (d) Itself

10. Zero divided by any number (except zero) gives _____.
    - (a) Zero
    - (b) One
    - (c) Two
    - (d) Three

11. Rahul has solved a division problem. Find out whether he has solved it correctly or not?
    $42 \div 8; Q = 5, R = 2$
    - (a) It is correct
    - (b) It is incorrect
    - (c) Can't say
    - (d) None of these

12. Solve the problem.
    $2663 \div 7$
    - (a) $Q = 380, R = 3$
    - (b) $Q = 380, R = 2$
    - (c) $Q = 380, R = 1$
    - (d) $Q = 383, R = 0$

13. Estimate the quotient.
    $256 \div 45$
    - (a) $Q = 5$
    - (b) $Q = 4$
    - (c) $Q = 3$
    - (d) $Q = 6$

14. Find the quotient and remainder.
    $93 \div 39$
    - (a) $Q = 2, R = 15$
    - (b) $Q = 3, R = 15$
    - (c) $Q = 1, R = 15$
    - (d) $Q = 15, R = 3$

15. A dozen has 12 units. How many dozens are there in 7044 units?
    - (a) 587
    - (b) 857
    - (c) 590
    - (d) 586

16. Find the divisor if dividend = 88, quotient = 12 and remainder = 4.
    - (a) 7
    - (b) 8
    - (c) 9
    - (d) 5

17. Find the dividend if divisor = 21, quotient = 43 and remainder = 19.
    (a) 920   (b) 922
    (c) 923   (d) 924

18. Complete the given pattern.
    $4 \div 2 = 2$
    $\_\_\_ \div 2 = 20$
    $400 \div 2 = \_\_\_$
    $4000 \div 2 = \_\_\_$
    (a) 40, 200, 2000
    (b) 400, 20, 200
    (c) 4, 200, 200
    (d) 4000, 200, 2000

19. Complete the given pattern.
    $8000 \div 4 = 2000$
    $_____ \div 40 = 200$
    $8000 \div 400 = \_\_\_\_$
    $_____ \div 4000 = 2$
    (a) 8000, 20, 8000
    (b) 8000, 200, 8000
    (c) 8000, 2000, 8000
    (d) 800, 200, 800

20. Solve the problem $518 \div 61$
    (a) Q = 8, R = 31
    (b) Q = 8, R = 30
    (c) Q = 8, R = 29
    (d) Q = 9, R = 30

21. There are 10 friends and 55 bananas. If the bananas are divided equally among the students, how many does each friend get?
    (a) Q = 5, R = 3   (b) Q = 5, R = 2
    (c) Q = 5, R = 5   (d) Q = 1, R = 5

22. Tina wants to buy 1250 cookies for a party. If there are 5 cookies in each package, how many packages should Tina buy?
    (a) 240   (b) 250
    (c) 260   (d) 125

23. A farmer picked 823 tomatoes from his field and divided them equally into 36 bunches. How many tomatoes are in each bunch? Is there any tomato left out from packing?
    (a) Q = 22, R = 31   (b) Q = 23, R = 32
    (c) Q = 21, R = 32   (d) Q = 31, R = 22

24. An ice cream vendor had 220 cherries. He split the cherries evenly among 110 ice cream sundaes. How many cherries did the vendor put on each sundae?
    (a) 3   (b) 4
    (c) 2   (d) 5

25. A group of 1500 students wants to ride a roller coaster. If the cars on the roller coaster can each hold 5 people, how many cars will students need?
    (a) 200   (b) 300
    (c) 400   (d) 500

☺☺☺

Factors and Multiples

Factors

If a given number is divisible by another number, then that number is a factor of the given number.

For example,

$28 = 1 \times 28, 28 = 4 \times 7, 28 = 2 \times 14$

So 1, 2, 4, 7, 14 and 28 are numbers each of which divides 28. We say 28 is divisible by 1, 2, 4, 7, 14 and 28. These are also called factors of 28.

Note: 1 and the number itself are factors of the given number.

For example, 3 and 4 are factors of 12, because $3 \times 4 = 12$.

Also $2 \times 6 = 12$ so 2 and 6 are also factors of 12.

And $1 \times 12 = 12$ so 1 and 12 are factors of 12 as well.

So all the factors of 12 are 1, 2, 3, 4, 6 and 12.

Note: A number can have many factors.

Example: Find out the factors of 6.

Solution: We have

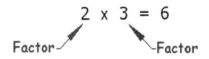

Thus, 2 and 3 are factors of 6.

Multiples

Multiples are products obtained by multiplying one number by another number.

For example, 8 and 11 are multiplied to get 88, So, 88 is a multiple of 8 and 11.

Factor Tree

Let us take an example of 24 to learn how to draw a factor tree.

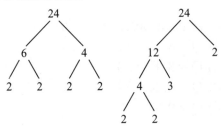

Thus, prime factors of 24 are 2 and 3.

Also, $24 = 3 \times 2 \times 2 \times 2$

Common Factors and Common Multiples

The factors or multiples that are common between two or more numbers are called common factors or multiples of given numbers.

For example, 5 is a factor of 35 as well as of 20. So 5 is a common factor of 35 and 20.

Clearly 1 is a common factor of every number.

Properties of Factors and Multiples

(i)   1 is a factor of every number.

(ii) Every number is a factor of itself.

(iii) Every factor of a number is an exact divisor of that number.

(iv) Factors of a given number are finite.

(v)   Prime numbers have only two factors: 1 and the number itself.

(vi) Every number is a multiple of itself.

(vii) Every multiple of a number is greater than or equal to that number.

(viii) The number of multiples of a given number is unlimited.

Prime Numbers

A number that has only two factors, that is 1 and the number itself is a prime number.

For example, 2, 3, 5, 7, 11, 13, are prime numbers.

Composite Numbers

Numbers which have more than two factors are called composite numbers. Composite numbers have atleast one factor other than 1 and the number itself.

For example, 4, 6, 8, 10, 12, are composite numbers.

Co-prime Numbers

Two different numbers which have no other common factor except 1 are called co-prime numbers.

For example, 12 and 25 have no common factor other than 1. So, 12 and 25 are co-prime numbers.

Highest Common Factor (HCF)

HCF of two or more numbers is the greatest common factor of the numbers.

Example: Find the HCF of 99 and 30.

Solution: $99 = 1 \times 99$

$\qquad = 3 \times 33$

$\qquad = 9 \times 11$

So, 1, 3, 9, 11, 33, and 99 are factors of 99.

$\qquad 30 = 1 \times 30$

$\qquad = 2 \times 15$

$\qquad = 3 \times 10$

$\qquad = 5 \times 6$

So, 1, 2, 3, 4, 5, 6, 10, 15 and 30 are factors of 30.

3 is the only common factor of 99 and 30.

Thus, HCF of 99 and 30 is 3.

Least Common Factor (LCM)

LCM of two or more numbers is the smallest common multiple of the given numbers.

Example: Find the LCM of 16 and 8.

Solution: Multiples of 16 are 16, 32, 48, ...

Multiples of 8 are 8, 16, 24, 32, ...

Common multiples are 16, 32, ...

Least common multiples is 16.

Thus, LCM of 16 and 8 is 16.

Multiple Choice Questions

1. Which one of the following is a factor of 45 and not a multiple of 3?
   (a) 5   (b) 9
   (c) 15   (d) 7

2. Which one of the following is a multiple of 2 but not a factor of 8?
   (a) 2   (b) 8
   (c) 4   (d) 6

3. Which is odd one out?
   (a) 26   (b) 39
   (c) 65   (d) 71

4. What are the multiples of 16 between 40 and 90?
   (a) 48, 64, 80
   (b) 44, 64, 80
   (c) 42, 66, 86
   (d) 46, 68, 88

5. What is seventh multiple of 9?
   (a) 81   (b) 56
   (c) 45   (d) 63

6. Find the missing numbers.

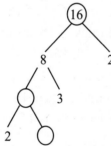

   (a) 2, 2   (b) 4, 2
   (c) 2, 3   (d) 3, 4

7. What is next number in the sequence?
   2, 6, 18, 54, ….
   (a) 216   (b) 162
   (c) 108   (d) 165

8. What is the greatest length that is used to measure 8 m, 6 m and 14 m exactly?
   (a) 4 m   (b) 3 m
   (c) 6 m   (d) 2 m

9. Which of the following numbers has the least number of factors?
   (a) 66   (b) 106
   (c) 78   (d) 110

10. Which of the numbers given below is a factor of 12?
   (a) 10   (b) 7
   (c) 5   (d) 6

11. Which of the numbers given below is not a factor of 8?
   (a) 3   (b) 2
   (c) 1   (d) 8

12. What is the HCF of 66 and 32?
   (a) 3   (b) 2
   (c) 4   (d) 6

13. Which is the smallest prime number?
   (a) 2   (b) 1
   (c) 3   (d) 5

14. What is the LCM of 18 and 24?
   (a) 24   (b) 36
   (c) 18   (d) 72

15. What is the first two common multiples of 2 and 5?
   (a) 10, 30   (b) 20, 30
   (c) 10, 20   (d) 10, 40

16. Which number is neither a prime nor a composite number?
   (a) 0   (b) 1
   (c) 2   (d) 4

17. Which number is an odd number?
   (a) 63   (b) 72
   (c) 64   (d) 56

18. Match the following:

	List I		List II
(i)	First 4 multiples of 3	A	6, 12, 18, 24
(ii)	First 4 multiples of 6	B	5, 10, 15, 20
(iii)	First 4 multiples of 5	C	10, 20, 30, 40
(iv)	First 4 multiples of 10	D	3, 6, 9, 12

	(i)	(ii)	(iii)	(iv)
(a)	A	B	C	D
(b)	D	A	B	C
(c)	B	C	A	D
(d)	D	B	C	A

19. From the list given below find how many numbers are factors of 125?

2, 3, 5, 7, 25, 50, 100

(a) 3 (b) 0

(c) 1 (d) 2

20. From the list given below find how many numbers are multiples of 20?

12, 25, 40, 36, 80, 100, 110, 150

(a) 3 (b) 0

(c) 1 (d) 2

21. A bell rings every 18 seconds, another every seconds. At 6:00 pm the two ring simultaneously. At what time will the bells ring again at the same time?

(a) 5 : 03 pm (b) 6 : 03 pm

(c) 6 : 05 pm (d) 6 : 59 pm

22. You are thinking of a number that is multiple of 7 and 12. What is the smallest number that you can think of?

(a) 168 (b) 49

(c) 84 (d) 36

23. There are 50 students on a field trip. The teacher thought of dividing the students in groups. Which of the following statements are true?

i. The teacher can make groups of 5

ii. The teacher can make groups of 10

iii. The teacher can make groups of 6

iv. The teacher can make groups of 7

(a) TTFF (b) FFTT

(c) TFTF (d) FTFT

24. Shraddha wants to buy flowers for her friends. She can buy roses in bunch of 7 flowers and carnations in bunch of 10 flowers. She wants to buy the same number of roses and carnations. What is the minimum number of flowers Shraddha will need to buy?

(a) 70 (b) 140

(c) 130 (d) 80

25. Sheetal has 45 green balls, 18 blue balls and 63 red balls. She wants to put them in bags with same number of each type of ball in each bag. How many bags will Sheetal need?

(a) 8 (b) 7

(c) 9 (d) 6

☺☺☺

Fractions

Learning Objectives:
In this chapter, students will learn about:
- Types of Fractions
- Lowest Form of Fractions
- Conversion of Fractions
- Addition, Subtraction, Multiplication and Division of Fractions

Fraction

We often say like half, one-fourth and three fourths.

For example,

(i) My mother gave me half a plate of rice.

(ii) I can drink only three-fourths of a glass of milk.

These terms show that they are parts of a whole. Fraction means 'a part of the whole'. In a fraction, the number above the horizontal line is the numerator and the number below the horizontal line is the denominator. For example, $\frac{1}{4}$, where 1 is the numerator and 4 is the denominator.

Types of Fractions

Like Fractions

Fractions which have the same denominator are called like fractions.

For example, $\frac{2}{3}$ and $\frac{1}{3}$ are like fractions.

Unlike Fractions

Fractions with different denominators are called unlike fractions.

For example, $\frac{2}{3}$ and $\frac{1}{5}$ are unlike fractions.

Proper Fractions

The fractions in which the numerator is less than the denominator are called proper fractions.

For example, $\frac{3}{4}$ and $\frac{4}{5}$. Its value is always less than 1

Improper Fractions

The fractions in which the numerator is greater than or equal to the denominator are called improper fractions.

For example, $\frac{4}{3}$ and $\frac{6}{5}$. Its value is always greater than or equal to 1.

Mixed Fractions

A fraction which consists of two parts, a whole number and a fraction is called mixed fraction.

For example, $3\frac{1}{2}$ and $6\frac{3}{4}$ are mixed fractions.

Equivalent Fractions

Some fractions may look different, but are really the same. For example,

4/8 (Four-Eighths) = 2/4 (Two-Quarters) = 1/2 (One-Half)

To get equivalent fractions for a given fraction, multiply its numerator and denominator by the same number.

Reducing a Fraction to its Lowest Term

A fraction is said to be in its lowest term if the numerator and denominator have only 1 as the common factor.

Example: Write $\dfrac{25}{20}$ to its lowest form.

Solution: $\dfrac{25}{20} = \dfrac{5}{4}$

So, $\dfrac{5}{4}$ is the lowest form of $\dfrac{25}{20}$

Comparing Fractions

The fraction with the greater numerator is the greater fraction.

Example: Arrange $\dfrac{1}{15}, \dfrac{2}{15}, \dfrac{4}{15}, \dfrac{8}{15}, \dfrac{19}{15}$ in ascending order.

Solution: On comparing the numerator we get, $2 < 4 < 8 < 11 < 19$ So, we have

$$\frac{2}{15} < \frac{4}{15} < \frac{8}{15} < \frac{11}{15} < \frac{19}{15}$$

This is the required ascending order.

Addition of Fractions

Adding Fractions with same Denominators

We can add fractions easily if denominator is the same:

1/4	1/4	2/4	1/2
(One-Quarter)	(One-Quarter)	(Two-Quarters)	(One-Half)

 + 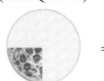 = =

Just add the numerators and write the sum over the same denominator.

Adding Fractions with Different Denominators

If the denominators are not the same, we make the denominators same.

1/3   1/6   ?

There are two ways to add fractions with different denominators:

(i) Common Denominator

One way is to multiply the given denominators together:

$$3 \times 6 = 18$$

Now, multiply $\dfrac{1}{3}$ by 6 and $\dfrac{1}{6}$ by 3.

We get, $\dfrac{1}{3} \times \dfrac{6}{6} = \dfrac{6}{18}$

and $\dfrac{1}{6} \times \dfrac{3}{3} = \dfrac{3}{18}$

So instead of having 3 or 6 slices, we will make both of them have 18 slices.

The pizzas now look like this (We will show calculations later):

6/18   3/18   9/18

(ii) Least Common Denominator

Another method is finding least common denominator.

Here is how to find out:

1/3	List the multiples of 3:	3, 6, 9, 12, 15, 18, 21, ...
1/6	List the multiples of 6:	6, 12, 18, 24, ...

Then find the smallest common multiple.

In the above we can see 6 is the smallest common multiple. So, the answer is 6.

So let us try using this methad. We want both to have 6 slices.

• When we multiply numerator and denominator of 1/3 by 2 we get 2/6.

• 1/6 already has a denominator of 6.

And our question now looks like:

2/6   1/6   3/6

Lastly we simplify it if possible. In this case 3/6 = 1/2.

Similarly we can subtract, divide and multiple fractions.

Converting an improper fraction into a mixed fraction

Example: Convert $\dfrac{15}{8}$ into a mixed fraction

Solution: On dividing 15 by 8 we get

Quotient = 1

Remainder = 7

Divisor = 8

Thus, $\dfrac{15}{8} = 1\dfrac{7}{8}$

Converting a mixed fraction into an improper fraction

Example: Convert $4\dfrac{1}{5}$ into an improper fraction.

Solution: $4\dfrac{1}{5} = \dfrac{4 \times 5 + 1}{5} = \dfrac{20 + 1}{5} = \dfrac{21}{5}$

Multiple Choice Questions

1. Pick the odd one out.
   (a) 3/8   (b) 4/9
   (c) 6/13   (d) 21/5

2. Write 31/8 as a mixed fraction.
   (a) 4   (b) 4(7/8)
   (c) 3(1/8)   (d) 3(7/8)

3. A fraction a/b = 1, when.
   (a) a > b   (b) a < b
   (c) a = b   (d) None of these

4. Convert 400 mL into L.
   (a) 4/10 L   (b) 3/10 L
   (c) 5/10 L   (d) 7/10 L

5. Pick the odd one out.
   (a) 2/5   (b) 3/5
   (c) 8/20   (d) 6/15

6. Which two fractions are equivalent?
   (a) 5/2 and 2/5
   (b) 4/3 and 8/6
   (c) 1/4 and 2/4
   (d) 2/3 and 1/3

7. Evaluate 5 2/3 − 3 1/2.
   (a) 2   (b) 2 (7/6)
   (c) 2 (1/6)   (d) 1 (2/5)

8. How many minutes are there in 2/3 of an hour?
   (a) 40 minutes   (b) 50 minutes
   (c) 60 minutes   (d) 20 minutes

9. If 1/3 + 1/6 + 1/12 = X, then X + 17/12
   = _____ .
   (a) 4   (b) 3
   (c) 2   (d) 1

10. Choose the incorrect option from the following.
    (a) 1/2 = 4/8   (b) 1/2 = 6/12
    (c) 1/3 = 5/10   (d) 1/3 = 5/15

11. What is the fraction used to represent the shaded parts?

    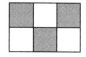

    (a) $\dfrac{3}{6} + \dfrac{4}{6}$ (b) $\dfrac{1}{6} + \dfrac{4}{6}$
    (c) $\dfrac{3}{6} + \dfrac{5}{6}$ (d) $\dfrac{3}{6} + \dfrac{1}{6}$

12. Reduce the given fraction to its lowest form. 9/15
    (a) 3/5   (b) 5/3
    (c) 3/15   (d) 5/9

Direction (13-16): Evaluate the following questions.

13. 2/5 × 3/4 × 5/8
    (a) 3/8   (b) 3/7
    (c) 3/16   (d) 6/20

14. 3/8 × 7/10 × 5/12
    (a) 7/64   (b) 7/81
    (c) 21/64   (d) 105/84

15. [2(1/2)] / [3(3)/4]
    (a) 8/75   (b) 1(1/2)
    (c) 2/3   (d) 9(3/8)

16. [3/8] / [5/12]
    (a) 1(1/9)   (b) 5/32
    (c) 4/5   (d) 9/10

17. The difference of shaded fraction of

    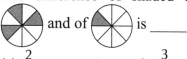

    (a) $\dfrac{2}{8}$ (b) $\dfrac{3}{8}$
    (c) $\dfrac{1}{8}$ (d) $\dfrac{5}{8}$

18. How many one-sixth will make one whole?
    (a) 6   (b) 3
    (c) 2   (d) 1

19. Arrange the following in ascending order?

$$\frac{5}{7}, \frac{9}{7}, \frac{3}{7}, \frac{1}{7}, \frac{4}{7}, \frac{10}{7}$$

(a) $\frac{4}{7}, \frac{3}{7}, \frac{1}{7}, \frac{5}{7}, \frac{9}{7}, \frac{10}{7}$

(b) $\frac{1}{7}, \frac{4}{7}, \frac{3}{7}, \frac{5}{7}, \frac{9}{7}, \frac{10}{7}$

(c) $\frac{1}{7}, \frac{3}{7}, \frac{4}{7}, \frac{5}{7}, \frac{9}{7}, \frac{10}{7}$

(d) $\frac{10}{7}, \frac{9}{7}, \frac{5}{7}, \frac{4}{7}, \frac{3}{7}, \frac{1}{7}$

19. Put >, < or = in the box.

$$\frac{2}{9} \square \frac{1}{7}$$

(a) >

(b) <

(c) =

(d) None of these

20. Convert $3\frac{4}{5}$ in improper fraction.

(a) $\frac{3}{5}$

(b) $\frac{19}{5}$

(c) $\frac{4}{5}$

(d) $\frac{17}{5}$

21. It takes Bhola 1/2 hour to wash, comb and put on his clothes and 1/4 hour to have his breakfast. How much time does it take Bhola to be ready for office?

(a) 3/4 hour

(b) 1 1/4 hour

(c) 2/4 hour

(d) 1 hour

22. Out of 20 people in a line for ice cream, one-quarter want vanilla. How many people want vanilla ice cream?

(a) 5

(b) 4

(c) 6

(d) 8

23. Out of 8 students in Mrs. Bhatia cart class, six-eights are in sixth grade. How many sixth graders are in Mrs. Bhatia's art class?

(a) 1

(b) 8

(c) 6

(d) 5

24. There are 12 berries in a bowl on the counter. Two-sixths of them are raspberries. How many raspberries are in the bowl?

(a) 5

(b) 8

(c) 4

(d) 6

25. Golu counted 8 students in the chair three-quarters of students have brown hair. How many students in the chair have brown hair?

(a) 4

(b) 5

(c) 6

(d) 7

☺☺☺

Measurement

Learning Objectives:
In this chapter, students will learn about:
- Length
- Weight
- Volume

Length

The standard unit for measuring length is metre.

We can also use centimetre and kilometre to measure the length of any object.

Length of cloth, the height of a wall, the height of a tree, the distance between two objects are all measured in metres. Carpenters use measuring tape for making furniture. Cloth merchant uses a metre rod for measuring length of clothes.

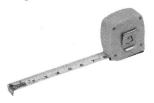

Measuring tape is also used by tailors for measuring length.

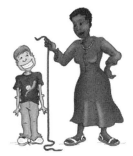

The metric system has prefix modifiers that are multiples of 10.

- 1 kilometre = 1000 metres
- 1 hectometre = 100 metres
- 1 decametre = 10 metres
- 1 decimetre = 1/10 metre
- 1 centimetre = 1/100 metre
- 1 millimetre = 1/1000 metre

As we move down the units, the next unit is one tenth as long. As we move upward, each unit is 10 times as long.

Notes:
- Always start from '0' while using measuring instruments.
- Millimetre (mm) and centimetre (cm) are used to measure small objects.
- Metre (m) is used to measure large objects.
- Metre (m) and kilometre (km) are used to measure large distances.
- Always convert the length of given objects into same unit of length before solving a problem.

Weight

The standard unit for measuring weight is kilogram. We weigh things in kilograms. Lighter objects and smaller quantities of things are weighed in grams. We write kilogram as kg and gram as gm.

A paperclip weighs about 1 gram.

We commonly see cast iron weights in vegetable shop which are used to measure weight of vegetables.

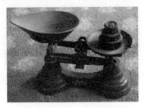

The metric system has prefix modifiers that are multiples of 10.

1 kilogram = 1000 grams

1 hectogram = 100 grams

1 decagram = 10 grams

1 decigram = 1/10 grams

1 centigram = 1/100 grams

1 millimetre = 1/1000 grams

Tonnes (also called Metric Tons) are used to measure things that are very heavy.

1 tonne = 1,000 kilograms

Things like cars, trucks and large cargo boxes are weighed using the tonne.

Notes:
- Always start from '0' while using weighing balance.
- Gram (gm) is used to weigh lighter objects.
- Kilogram (kg) is used to measure heavier objects.
- Always convert the weight of given objects into same unit of weight before adding or subtracting them.

Volume

The capacity or volume of a container is the maximum amount of liquid which it can hold. The standard unit for measuring capacity is litre.

The metric system has prefix modifiers that are multiples of 10.

- 1 kilolitre = 1000 litres
- 1 hectolitre = 100 litres
- 1 decilitre = 10 litres
- 1 decilitre = 1/10 litre
- 1 centilitre = 1/100 litre
- 1 millilitre = 1/1000 litre

As we move down the units, the next unit is one tenth as large. As we move upward, each unit is 10 times as large. One hundred millilitres, which is 1/10 litre (100/1000 = 1/10) are larger than one centilitre (1/100th litre).

Notes:
- Always use a container of capacity 1 litre to find the capacity of other containers
- To find the volume of a liquid, just pour it in a container with a measuring scale marked on it.
- Millilitre is used to measure less quantity of liquid.
- Litre is used to measure greater quantity of liquid.
- Always convert the volumes of given liquid into same unit of volume before adding or subtracting them.

Multiple Choice Questions

Direction (1-5): Read the data given below and answer the questions:

Giraffe	Height of Giraffe
A.	438 cm
B.	620 cm
C.	286 cm
D.	526 cm

1. Which is the tallest Giraffe?
   (a) D   (b) C
   (c) B   (d) A

2. How much taller is Giraffe B than A?
   (a) 180 cm   (b) 181 cm
   (c) 182 cm   (d) 183 cm

3. How much shorter is Giraffe C than D?
   (a) 210 cm   (b) 220 cm
   (c) 230 cm   (d) 240 cm

4. Which is the shortest Giraffe?
   (a) D   (b) C
   (c) B   (d) A

5. How much taller is the tallest Giraffe than the shortest Giraffe?
   (a) 331 cm   (b) 332 cm
   (c) 333 cm   (d) 334 cm

6. 77 km + 2 m + 99 km 5 m = _____
   (a) 176 km   (b) 166 km 47 m
   (c) 176 km 46 m   (d) 176 km 40 m

7. $\boxed{1000 \text{ m}}$ = _____

   (a) $\boxed{50 \text{ m}}$ $\boxed{50 \text{ m}}$ $\boxed{800 \text{ m}}$

   (b) $\boxed{500 \text{ m}}$ $\boxed{250 \text{ m}}$ $\boxed{250 \text{ m}}$

   (c) $\boxed{250 \text{ m}}$ $\boxed{250 \text{ m}}$ $\boxed{250 \text{ m}}$

   (d) $\boxed{900 \text{ m}}$ $\boxed{50 \text{ m}}$ $\boxed{25 \text{ m}}$

8. Find the longest item from the given table.

Items	Lengths
Notebook	70 cm
Pencil	0.15 m
Pen	160 mm
Brush	20 cm

   (a) Brush   (b) Pen
   (c) Pencil   (d) Notebook

9. Find the difference between 65 L 534 mL and 32 L 876 mL.
   (a) 30 L 870 mL
   (b) 32 L 658 mL
   (c) 31 L 658 mL
   (d) 30 L 670 mL

10. Convert 33340 mL into Litres and millilitres.
   (a) 33 L 350 mL
   (b) 333 L 40 mL
   (c) 30 L 340 mL
   (d) 33 L 340 mL

11. Shraddha has written following statements about the metric unit she would use to measure some objects. Find the incorrect sentence among them:

    i. Centimetre is used to measure the length of a pencil.

    ii. Kilometre is used to measure distance from a city to another.

    iii. Metre is used to measure depth of a bucket.

    iv. Metre is used to measure height of a tree.

    (a) ii   (b) ii

    (c) iv   (d) i

12. 25 L 850 mL and 19 L 390 mL.

    (a) 45 L 240 mL

    (b) 46 L 245 mL

    (c) 40 L 240 mL

    (d) 45 L 290 mL

13. $1 \text{ mg} = \dfrac{1}{1000}$ _____.

    (a) mg   (b) g

    (c) hg   (d) dag

14. 19677 m = 19 km + _____ m

    (a) 77   (b) 600

    (c) 677   (d) 500

15. 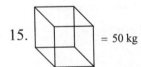 = 50 kg

Choose the measure that ads up to the measure of the cube.

    (a) | 4 kg | + | 1 kg | + | 20 kg | + | 30 kg |

    (b) | 20 kg | + | 20 kg | + | 20 kg |

    (c) | 25 kg | + | 25 kg |

    (d) | 50000 g |

16. 4300 m = 4000 m + 300 m = _____ km _____ m

    (a) 4000, 300   (b) 40, 300

    (c) 4, 300   (d) 400, 300

17. Add 95 cm 5 mm and 97 cm 5 mm.

    (a) 192 cm 10 mm

    (b) 190 cm 10 mm

    (c) 193 cm

    (d) 180 cm

18. The sum of each row and column is given below.

Pen	Flower Pot	Pen	45 cm
Book	Flower Pot	Pen	85 cm
Book	Book	Pen	110 cm
110 cm	100 cm	30 cm	

    What is the length of flower pot?

    (a) 25 cm   (b) 50 cm

    (c) 10 cm   (d) 85 cm

19. If weight of 8 identical balls = 2000 g, then weight of each identical ball = ___ g.

    (a) 100   (b) 200

    (c) 250   (d) 500

20. Which of the following options is incorrect?

    (a) 2 km 90 m = 2090 m

    (b) 2 km 58 m = 2058 m

    (c) 3 km 80 m = 3800 m

    (d) 6 km 1 m = 6001 m

21. A carpenter was making a shelf. Shelf needed to be 86 cm long but piece of wood he had was 1 m and 26 m long. His saw was 33 cm long. How much did he have to cut off the piece of wood to make it fit?

    (a) 40 cm   (b) 43 cm

    (c) 50 cm   (d) 53 cm

22. A container has 2550 mL of water. How many litres and millilitres of water is in the container?
    (a) 2 L 50
    (b) 2 L 525 mL
    (c) 2 L 5(

23. Rohan b
    used 44
    is left?
    (a) 5 I
    (c) 5

24. A jar can hold 4 L 250 mL honey. How much honey will be needed to fill 4 jars?
    (a) 16 litres
    (b) 15 litres
    (c) 17 litres
    (d) 17 L 250 mL

25. If the cost of 1 litre of cough syrup is ₹ 480. 40, find the cost of 500 mL.
    (a))0.40
    (b) ₹ 220.40
    (c) 60.40
    (d) ₹ 240.20

1008
9789357940535
1008

Location: 2-A

BBM 2W2Y

Title:
International Maths Olympiad - Class 4 with CD. Theories with Examples, Mcqs and Solutions, Previ...

Cond: Very Good
User: mcsales
Station: MF-North
Date: 2025-02-20 05.49.52 (UTC)
count: Benjamins Bookshelf
Loc: 2-A
BBM 2W2Y
BBV 9357940537.VG
1008
26773847
0 36 in
083,600

3V 9357940537.VG

Money

Money

Money is any object or record that is generally accepted as payments for goods and services.

Unit of Currency in India

The unit of currency in India is Rupees.

    1 rupee = 100 paise

The paper based notes available in India are of ₹ 1000, ₹ 500, ₹ 100, ₹ 50, ₹ 20, ₹ 5 as shown below:

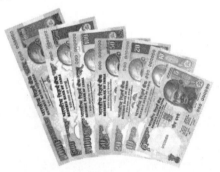

Few important currencies of the world are United States – Dollars, UK Pound – Sterling and Euro.

The coins available in India for circulation are of ₹ 10, ₹ 5, ₹ 2 and ₹ 1 as shown below:

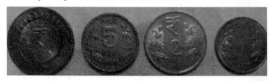

When one goes to market to purchase and gives more money than the price of material, then the shopkeeper will return the money back. That returned money is known as change.

Misconcept/Concept

Misconcept: If a paper note is mutilated or torn, then you lose money as you feel that it cannot be used as no shopkeeper is ready to take it.

Concept: Mutilated notes can be tendered at all bank branches for the exchange obtained. Payment exchange value of mutilated notes is governed by the Reserve Bank of India (Note Refund) Rules and one can get full/ half/no value depending on the condition of the note.

Multiple Choice Questions

1. Two pens cost ₹ 24. Find the cost of 5 such pens.
   (a) ₹ 40   (b) ₹ 50
   (c) ₹ 60   (d) ₹ 70

2. Add ₹ 150.60 and ₹ 140.75 and then subtract the obtained sum from ₹ 325.50.
   (a) ₹ 32.75   (b) ₹ 34.15
   (c) ₹ 33.25   (d) ₹ 34.75

Direction (3-6): Consider the prices of the items below to answer question.

Apple --------- ₹ 180 per kg

Pen --------- ₹ 8 per piece

Eraser ------- ₹ 5 for 2 erasers

Chocolates ------- ₹ 15 for 3 chocolates

3. Ankit wants to buy half kg apples and one chocolate. The total amount he needs to pay is _____.
   (a) ₹ 85   (b) ₹ 95
   (c) ₹ 90   (d) ₹ 105

4. If Bunny wants to buy one pen and 3 erasers, how much he needs to pay?
   (a) ₹ 13   (b) ₹ 15
   (c) ₹ 15.50   (d) ₹ 16.25

5. One kg apples can be bought for ₹ 180 and two chocolates can be bought for ₹ 7.50. This statement is _____.
   (a) True
   (b) False
   (c) Insufficient information
   (d) None of these

6. If Manpreet has ₹ 122 and he wants to buy as many chocolates as he can with this amount. The number of chocolates that he can buy is _____.
   (a) 15   (b) 20
   (c) 24   (d) 30

7. Multiply ₹ 435.60 by 12.
   (a) ₹ 5227.20
   (b) ₹ 6227.20
   (c) ₹ 5227
   (d) ₹ 5127.01

8. Yuvraj is very fond of reading books. Once he bought books for ₹ 465 and she paid ₹ 500 to the bookstore, which expression shows the correct amount of change that he will get back?
   (a) ₹ 500 + ₹ 465
   (b) ₹ 500 − ₹ 465
   (c) ₹ 500 ÷ ₹ 465
   (d) ₹ 500 × ₹ 465

Direction(9-12): Consider the following scenario to answer questions.

Shraddha and Shubhra are two friends and one day they decided to go to shopping together. Shraddha had ₹ 1500 and Shubhra had ₹ 2000 with them. Shraddha purchased shoes for ₹ 550, a skirt for ₹ 275 and movie DVD for ₹ 50. Shubhra purchased a top for ₹ 250, a bag for ₹ 480, a book for ₹ 115 and a tennis racket for ₹ 500.

9. What is the total money spent by Shraddha and Shubhra together in shopping?
   (a) ₹ 2220   (b) ₹ 2170
   (c) ₹ 1720   (d) ₹ 880

10. The amount left with Shubhra after shopping is _____.
   (a) ₹ 540   (b) ₹ 550
   (c) ₹ 555   (d) ₹ 655

11. On the way back to home, Shraddha purchased a toy for his little brother worth ₹ 99. Now how much money is left with her?
   (a) ₹ 426   (b) ₹ 476
   (c) ₹ 526   (d) ₹ 626

12. If the amount left with Shubhra is to be divided equally into 5 parts, what will be amount of one part?
    (a) ₹ 108   (b) ₹ 110
    (c) ₹ 111   (d) ₹ 131

Direction (13-14): Consider the following scenario to answer the questions.

The sum of money with Ankit and Golu is equal to the money with Sheetal. The total money with all three of them is ₹ 150.

13. How much money is present with Sheetal?
    (a) ₹ 35   (b) ₹ 50
    (c) ₹ 60   (d) ₹ 75

14. The amount of money present with Golu is _____.
    (a) ₹ 25
    (b) ₹ 40
    (c) ₹ 75
    (d) Data insufficient

15. How much money is needed to add to ₹ 525.50 to get ₹ 1000?
    (a) ₹ 475.50   (b) ₹ 473.25
    (c) ₹ 474.25   (d) ₹ 474.50

16. What is the difference between 745 rupees 35 paise and 178 rupees 59 paise?
    (a) ₹ 566.76   (b) ₹ 567
    (c) ₹ 565.50   (d) ₹ 566.75

17. If the cost of 250 g of potatoes is ₹ 20, then what is the cost of 2 kg of potatoes?
    (a) ₹ 160   (b) ₹ 180
    (c) ₹ 190   (d) ₹ 150

18. The following is the bill of fruits bought by Naresh from a shop?

Items	Cost
Apple	₹ 140
Orange	₹ 90
Grapes	₹ 70

If Naresh paid ₹ 1000, then how much will he get back?
    (a) ₹ 650   (b) ₹ 810
    (c) ₹ 700   (d) ₹ 750

19. Two kg sugar cost ₹ 50. Find the cost of 10 kg sugar.
    (a) ₹ 200   (b) ₹ 225
    (c) ₹ 250   (d) ₹ 300

20. 10 teachers decide to buy a gift for their principal. If the price of gift is ₹ 500, what will be the share of one teacher?
    (a) ₹ 50   (b) ₹ 60
    (c) ₹ 75   (d) ₹ 100

21. Sohans father needs to pay ₹ 3000 for Sohan quarterly school fees. He has the following amount with him. How much more amount he needs so that he can pay ₹ 3000 as quarterly fees?
    i.   1 note of ₹ 1000
    ii. 2 notes of ₹ 500
    iii. 4 note of ₹ 100
    iv. 7 notes of ₹ 50
    v.   3 notes of ₹ 20
    (a) ₹ 150   (b) ₹ 590
    (c) ₹ 250   (d) ₹ 190

22. Ashu's father returned from a foreign trip and brought with him some currencies like 10 notes of US dollars, 5 notes of 10 UK pounds. If the price of 1 US Dollar = ₹ 50 and price of 1 UK pound = ₹ 80, then the total amount in ₹ that he has is _____
    (a) ₹ 14000
    (b) ₹ 900
    (c) ₹ 10000
    (d) ₹ 4000

23. A family of four i.e. father, mother and two children went to visit a zoo and took ₹ 1000 with them. The cost of zoo ticket is ₹ 50 per adult and ₹ 20 per child. They spent ₹ 200 for food and ₹ 50 to purchase bananas for monkeys. What is the total amount family spent during the visit?

(a) ₹ 320   (b) ₹ 390

(c) ₹ 400   (d) None of these

24. Swati is very fond of collecting different kinds of currencies both coins and paper notes. She has coins of 10 p, 25 p, 50 p, ₹ 1, ₹ 5, ₹ 10, and notes of ₹ 5 ₹ 10, ₹ 20, ₹ 50, and ₹ 100. What is the total amount of money with her?

(a) ₹ 195.75   (b) ₹ 201.85

(c) ₹ 200.75   (d) ₹ 200.85

25. Rajesh needs to buy an ice-cream worth ₹ 10. He has some coins of 25p, 50 p, and ₹ 1. Which of the following combination of coins will help him in buying the ice-cream?

(a) 8 coins of 25 p, 6 coins of 50 p, and 6 coins of ₹ 1.

(b) 2 coins of 25 p, 12 coins of 50 p and 4 coins of ₹ 1.

(c) 8 coins of 25 p, 4 coins of 50 p and 5 coins of ₹ 1.

(d) 4 coins of 25 p, 8 coins of 50 p and 5 coins of ₹ 1.

Time and Calendar

Learning Objectives:

In this chapter, students will learn about:

- Clock and Time
- Months, weeks and days in Calendar

Time

Time is a measure for events that are happening now or that had happened before.

Like length, weight or height have units, Time also has units. These are years, months weeks, days, hours, minutes and seconds.

To measure with hours, minutes and seconds, we use clock. In a day we have 24 hours.

Clock and Time

A clock dial has 60 divisions. These divisions show minutes and seconds. There are 12 numerals marked from 1 to 12 on clock face which are at an equal distances.

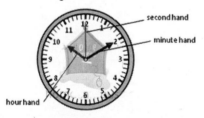

5th division, 5th is marked with 1, 10th division with 2 and so are 15th, 20th, 25th, 30th, 35th, 40th, 50th, 55th, and 60th, divisions marked with 3, 4, 5, 6, 7, 8, 9, 10, 11 and 12, respectively. These divisions, generally shown with longer lines than other divisions, represent hours.

The minute hand takes 60 seconds in moving from one division to next division. This is known as 1 minute.

60 seconds = 1 minute

The minute hand takes 5 minutes in reaching from one marked numeral to next marked numeral. And in completing one full revolution it takes 60 minutes. This is called one hour.

60 minutes = 1 hour

An hour hand moves from one numeral to next numeral in 60 minutes.

Further we have second hand which takes 1 minute to complete one round.

60 seconds = 1 minute

Calendar

There are many ways of measuring time in months, weeks or days and that is called a calendar. We have 12 months namely January, February, March, April, May, June, July, August, September, October, November, December. Some months have 30 days and some have 31 days. February is a month where we have 28 days but every leap year we have February with 29 days.

Further 7 days make a week. Name of the days are:

Sunday, Monday, Tuesday, Wednesday, Thursday, Friday, Saturday

Following is the calendar of the June month of year 2014:

June 2018						
Sunday	Monday	Tuesday	Wednesday	Thursday	Friday	Saturday
					1	2
3	4	5	6	7	8	9
10	11	12	13	14	15	16
17	18	19	20	21	22	23
24	25	26	27	28	29	30

We read the calendar to tell the days and dates. For example, from above calendar 9th June falls on Saturday.

A date is written as follows:

Date/month/year, example: 14/06/2018

Or

Date-month-year, example: 14-06-2108

Or

Date month' year, example: 14th June' 2018

Multiple Choice Questions

1. Pick the odd one out.
   - (a) January
   - (b) July
   - (c) May
   - (d) November

2. Today is Monday. After 61 days, it will be _____.
   - (a) Wednesday
   - (b) Saturday
   - (c) Tuesday
   - (d) Thursday

3. The difference between 7 hours 25 min and 3 hrs 45 min is _____.
   - (a) 4 hrs 15 min
   - (b) 4 hrs 65 min
   - (c) 3 hrs 40 min
   - (d) 4 hrs 45 min

4. The time from 12 mid night to 12 noon is noted as _____.
   - (a) am
   - (b) pm
   - (c) midnight
   - (d) day

5. PM means _____.
   - (a) post meridian
   - (b) post noon
   - (c) pre noon
   - (d) none of these

6. 3 hrs 33 min = _____ min.
   - (a) 333
   - (b) 210
   - (c) 213
   - (d) 180

7. How many weeks are there in 1 year?
   - (a) 55
   - (b) 53
   - (c) 51
   - (d) 52

8. The month with neither 31 days nor 30 days is _____.
   - (a) February
   - (b) April
   - (c) November
   - (d) December

9. What does am stands for?
   - (a) After noon
   - (b) Before noon
   - (c) Midnight
   - (d) None of these

10. Which of the following is a leap year?
    - (a) 2011
    - (b) 2013
    - (c) 2015
    - (d) 2016

11. 5 years 3 months = _____
    - (a) 70 months
    - (b) 63 months
    - (c) 54 months
    - (d) 46 months

12. How many years are between 1956 and 1999?
    - (a) 34 years
    - (b) 43 years
    - (c) 54 years
    - (d) 31 years

13. How many days are in 60 weeks?
    - (a) 400
    - (b) 420
    - (c) 300
    - (d) 450

14. Put >, < or = in the following.
    44 months _____ 3 years
    - (a) <
    - (b) >
    - (c) =
    - (d) Cann't say

15. 6 days = ____ hours
    - (a) 100
    - (b) 120
    - (c) 140
    - (d) 144

16. Half an hour is ____ minutes.
    - (a) 30
    - (b) 60
    - (c) 45
    - (d) 15

17. Choose the correct time '20 minutes after 2:15'.
    - (a) 1:55
    - (b) 2:45
    - (c) 2:35
    - (d) 2:45

18. Which is the most likely time to eat lunch?
    - (a) 2:00 p.m.
    - (b) 7:00 a. m.
    - (c) 11:00 a. m.
    - (d) 8:00 p.m.

19. What does quarter part two means?
    - (a) 2:15
    - (b) 2:30
    - (c) 2:40
    - (d) 2:45

20. Find the start if elapsed time is 2 hours and 20 minutes and finish time is 3 : 40 a.m.
    - (a) 1:20 a.m.
    - (b) 1:20 p.m.
    - (c) 2:20 a.m.
    - (d) 2:20 p.m.

21. Aditya spent 25 minutes on his home work last night. He started it at 9: 50 pm. On what time did he finish his homework?
   (a) 9:15   (b) 10:15
   (c) 9:10   (d) 10:10

22. Ali took 54 minutes to walk to school. Her brother took 18 minutes less to walk to the same school. How long did it take Ali brother to walk to school?
   (a) 30 min   (b) 36 min
   (c) 38 min   (d) 35 min

23. The Khurana family is going to see a movie at 5:50 pm. It is 11:20 am right now. How long do they have to wait to see the movie?
   (a) 5 hour 20 min
   (b) 6 and a half hours
   (c) 6 hours
   (d) 6 hours 20 minutes

24. Ayushi slept from 9:00 pm until 7:00 am. She had a bad dream and could not sleep from 2:45 am until 3:30 am. How many hours did she sleep?
   (a) 10 and half an hours
   (b) 11 hours 45 minutes
   (c) 9 hours 15 minutes
   (d) 9 hours 45 minutes

25. Tina and Mina are traveling to New York city. Tina's plane arrives at 8:00 am but Mina's plane arrives 2 hours and 30 minutes later to Tinas plane. What time does Mina's plane arrive?
   (a) 8:30 am
   (b) 9:30 am
   (c) 10:30 am
   (d) 11:30 am

Geometry

> **Learning Objectives:**
> In this chapter, students will learn about:
> - Plane Geometry
> - Open Figure
> - Closed Figure
> - Symmetry

Plane Geometry

A plane is a flat, two dimensional surface. It deals with shapes like lines, circles, triangles, square, etc.

Point

A point represents a position in space. It is represented by a small dot.

Line

A straight path on a plane extending in both directions with no end points, is called a line.

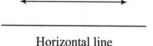

Horizontal line

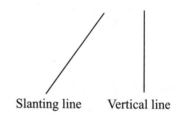

Slanting line   Vertical line

Line segment

It is the part of a line that has two end points. Thus, it has a definite length.

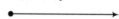

Ray

A line segment extended indefinitely in one direction is called a ray.

Type of Lines

Definition	What You Draw	What You Say	What You Write
Parallel Lines stay the same distance apart and never touch.	A B C D	Line AB is parallel to line CD.	$\overleftrightarrow{AB} \parallel \overleftrightarrow{DC}$
Intersecting Lines meet or cross each other.	A D C B	Line AB intersects line CD.	$\overleftrightarrow{AB}$ intersects $\overleftrightarrow{DC}$

Perpendicular Lines are lines that meet or cross and form right angles.	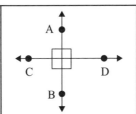	Line AB is perpendicular to line CD.	$\overleftrightarrow{AB} \perp \overleftrightarrow{DC}$

Polygon

A polygon is a two-dimensional object in a plane with enclosed sides. The number of sides of a polygon determines the type of polygon.

The simplest form of a polygon is a triangle.

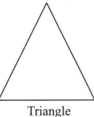

Triangle

Regular Polygon: In this type of polygons, all the sides have equal length and all the angles have equal measure.

For example:

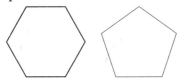

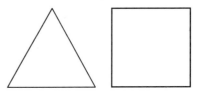

Irregular Polygon: In this type of polygons, all the sides don't have equal length and all the angles don't have equal measure.

For example:

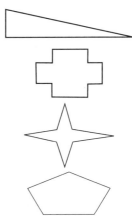

Some examples of polygon are:

Triangle	Quadrilateral	Pentagon	Hexagon	Octagon
3 sides	4 sides	5 sides	6 sides	8 sides
3 angles	4 angles	5 angles	6 angles	8 angles

Types of Triangles

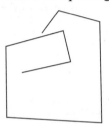	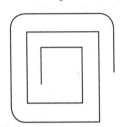	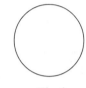
Scalene Triangle	Isosceles Triangle	Equilateral Triangle
No sides are equal	Two sides are equal	All sides are equal

Open Figure

If a figure starts and ends at the same point, it is called an open figure. For example:

Closed Figure

If a figure does not has same starting and ending point, it is called a closed figure. For example:

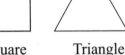

Square   Triangle   Circle

Types of Quadrilaterals

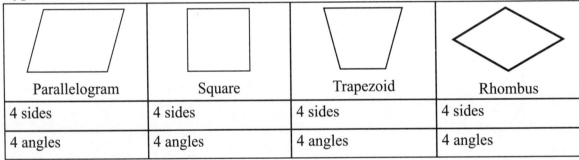

Parallelogram	Square	Trapezoid	Rhombus
4 sides	4 sides	4 sides	4 sides
4 angles	4 angles	4 angles	4 angles

Perimeter

Perimeter is used to describe the distance around the boundary of an object or shape. To find the perimeter of any shape, add the lengths of its sides.

Example: Shraddha's backyard is 100 feet in length and 50 feet in width. Find the perimeter of the backyard.

Solution: Required perimeter = 100 + 100 + 50 + 50 = 300 feet

Example: Think of yourself walking around the boundary of a barn. The length of the barn is 75 feet and the width of the barn is 90 feet. Find the perimeter.

Solution: Perimeter of the barn
= 75 + 90 + 75 + 90 = 330 feet

Area

Area is the number of square units needed to cover a flat surface. Some metric units for measuring area are square centimetre, square decimetre, or square metre.

Let us find the area of the given figures by counting the squares.

1 square unit

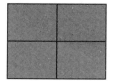

4 square units

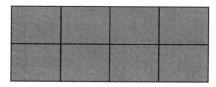

8 square units

Now we are finding the area of shaded squares of the given figures.

1 square cm

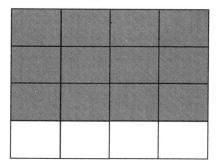

12 square cm

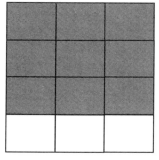

9 square cm

Sometimes we need to count half squares to find the area of a figure.

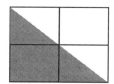

1 whole square + 2 half squares

Also,   2 half squares = 1 whole square

So,   1 + 1 = 2 square units

Sometimes we need to estimate the area of a figure.

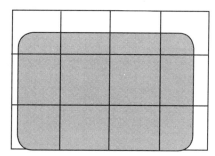

4 whole squares + 4 almost whole squares + 4 about half squares

Now,   4 half squares = 2 whole squares

4 + 4 + 2 = 10 square units

Square

A square has four sides and four corners. Also, all the sides of a square are equal.

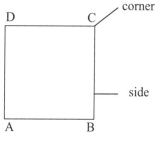

Square

Area of a square = (side)^2

Perimeter of a square = side + side + side + side

= 4 × side

Rectangle

A rectangle has four sides and four corners. Also, the opposite sides of a rectangle are equal.

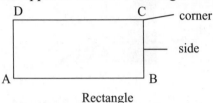

Rectangle

Area of a rectangle
= AB × BC = Length × Breadth
Perimeter of a rectangle
= 2 (Length + Breadth) = 2 [AB + BC]

Circle

A circle has no sides and no corners. It is a closed shape.

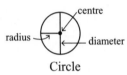

Circle

In a circle the length of diameter = 2 × the length of radius
or Radius = diameter of circle/2

Drawing a Circle

Steps to draw a circle by using compass are:
Step 1: Keep the compass pointed end on paper.
Step 2: Now, stretch the other end having arm without disturbing the pointed end of compass.

Three-dimensional Shapes

Three-dimensional shapes or 3D shapes have three measurements that is length, breadth and height.
Face: A face is a surface or flat side of a solid.
Edge: It is the line segment where two faces of a solid meet.
Vertex: It is the point where three or more faces meet.

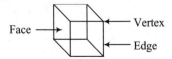

Cube

A cube has 6 faces, 12 faces and 8 vertices.

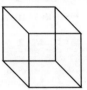

Cuboid

A cuboid has 6 faces, 12 faces and 8 vertices.

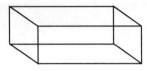

Cone

A cone has 2 faces (1 flat and 1 curved), 1 edge and 1 vertex.

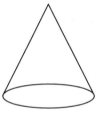

Cylinder

A cylinder has 3 faces (2 flat and 1 curved), edges and no vertex.

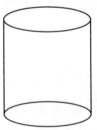

Sphere

A sphere has 1 curved surface, no edge and no vertex.

Symmetry

When one shape becomes exactly like another if you flip, slide or turn it this is called symmetry

The figure in which one part overlaps with the other part exactly, the figures are called symmetrical.

Reflection Symmetry

The simplest symmetry is Reflection Symmetry (sometimes called Line Symmetry or Mirror Symmetry). It is easy to see, because one half is the reflection of the other half. Here a dog has her face made perfectly symmetrical with a bit of photo magic. The white line down the center is the Line of Symmetry.

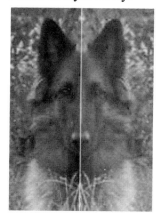

The Line of Symmetry does not have to be up-down or left-right, it can be in any direction.

Rotational Symmetry

With Rotational Symmetry, the image is rotated around a central point so that it appears 2 or more times. The number of times it appears is called the Order.

Here are some examples.

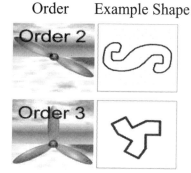

Order   Example Shape

Point Symmetry

Point Symmetry is when every part has a matching part.

(i) the same distance from the central point.

(ii) but in the opposite direction.

It is also the same as "Rotational Symmetry of Order 2" as discussed above.

Net

A net of a 3D shape can be obtained by unfolding the shape.

For example, Net of a cube

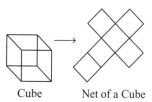

Cube   Net of a Cube

Multiple Choice Questions

1. What do we call a six-sided polygon?
   - (a) Heptagon
   - (b) Henagon
   - (c) Hexagon
   - (d) Pentagon

2. How many rectangles are there in the following picture?

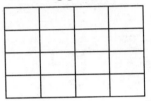

   - (a) 23
   - (b) 24
   - (c) 25
   - (d) 16

3. Some shapes can be fitted together, edge to edge. This is called _____.
   - (a) Paper folding
   - (b) Tiling
   - (c) Paper cutting
   - (d) Tangrams

4. The distance between the centre and any point on the circle is called its.
   - (a) Radius
   - (b) Diameter
   - (c) Circumference
   - (d) Area

5. The perimeter of the circle is called its _____.
   - (a) Radius
   - (b) Diameter
   - (c) Circumference
   - (d) Centre

6. How many triangles are there in the given figure.

   - (a) 15
   - (b) 13
   - (c) 16
   - (d) 12

7. Which of the following dotted liens represents the line of symmetry?

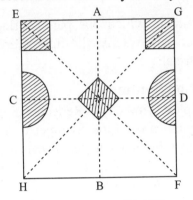

   - (a) GH
   - (b) EF
   - (c) CD
   - (d) AB

8. What is the perimeter of the given figure?

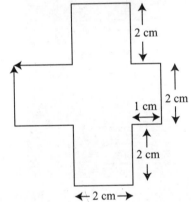

   - (a) 20 cm
   - (b) 15 cm
   - (c) 12 cm
   - (d) 22 cm

9. Which of the following figures has highest area?

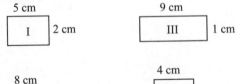

   - (a) I
   - (b) II
   - (c) III
   - (d) IV

10. Which of the following figures has exactly 3 faces?

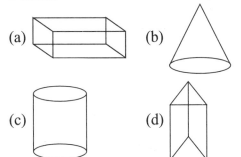

(a)   (b)

(c)   (d)

11. Name the figure obtained on joining the given three points.

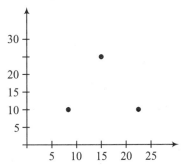

(a) Line   (b) Triangle
(c) Square   (d) Quadrilateral

12. If perimeter of 1 small square is 4 m then what is the area of the whole given figure?

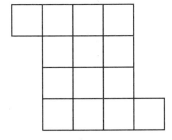

(a) 14 square metre
(b) 15 square metre
(c) 16 square metre
(d) 17 square metre

13. If the side of an equilateral triangle is 10 cm, then find the perimeter of triangle.
(a) 80 cm   (b) 50 cm
(c) 25 cm   (d) 30 cm

14. What is the perimeter of square of side 9 cm?
(a) 35 cm   (b) 36 cm
(c) 37 cm   (d) 38 cm

15. What is the area of 11 unit squares?
(a) 110 square units
(b) 100 square units
(c) 11 square units
(d) 10 square units

16. Metre is the unit of _____.
(a) Area   (b) Volume
(c) Perimeter   (d) Rupees

Direction (17-20): Shraddha is making bed-sheets to sell it in the market. She makes bed-sheets of different sizes. The table showing size and price of the bedsheet is given below. Read and answer the questions that follow.

S. No.	Bedsheet	Length	Width	Price
1	Small	2 m	1 m	₹ 100
2	Medium	3 m	2 m	₹ 200
3	Large	4 m	3 m	₹ 300
4	Extra large	5 m	4 m	₹ 400
5	Deluxe	6 m	5 m	₹ 500

17. A customer asked for two extra large bedsheets. What is the perimeter of each bedsheet?
(a) 17 m   (b) 18 m
(c) 36 m   (d) 34 m

18. What is the difference between the perimeter of medium bedsheets and deluxe bedsheets?
(a) 10 m   (b) 11 m
(c) 12 m   (d) 13 m

19. A customer asked for 2 small bedsheets, 1 large bedsheet and 2 deluxe bedsheets. How much did he/she have to pay?
(a) ₹ 1000   (b) ₹ 1500
(c) ₹ 2000   (d) ₹ 2500

20. What is the difference between the perimeter of large bedsheet and small bedsheet?

    (a) 5 m   (b) 6 m

    (c) 7 m   (d) 8 m

21. Mr. Kumar bought a rectangular field whose length is thrice its breadth. If the breadth of the field is 50 m, find the boundary of the field.

    (a) 400 m   (b) 350 m

    (c) 450 m   (d) 380 m

22. Neha made a box by folding the given cardboard along the dotted lines.

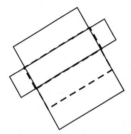

    (a) Sphere   (b) Cylinder

    (c) Cone   (d) Cuboid

23. Kiran walked along the boundry of a square-shaped park that has 20 m as its side. Rahul walked along the boundary of a rectangular-shaped park that has

20 m × 10 m as its dimension.

Find who walked more.

    (a) Rahul

    (b) Kiran

    (c) Both walked same distance

    (d) Cann't say

24. Rohan cut a piece of paper with 5 sides. What is the shape of the paper?

    (a) Triangle

    (b) Quadrilateral

    (c) Square

    (d) Pentagon

48. Naina, Shonam, Sohail and Tanu have a circular bangle of radius 2 cm, 3 cm, 5 cm, 1 cm, respectively.

Who has largest bangle?

    (a) Sohail   (b) Shonam

    (c) Naina   (d) Tanu

Pictorial Representation of Data

Learning Objectives:

In this chapter, students will learn about:

- Data
- Pictograph
- Bar Graph
- Pie Chart

Data

Data is facts that are collected by counting things, objects or events.

Data handling is a process of collection and representation of data in various forms.

Tally Mark

Tally marks are vertical lines. Here are the tally marks for 1 to 4:

  1   2   3   4

The 5th mark is drawn across the previous 4 marks:

5

Then continue making single marks again:

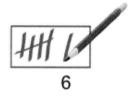

6

Note: Every fifth mark is drawn across the previous 4 marks.

Example: A tally of 12

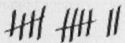

We can see there are two 5s (making 10) plus another 2 singles, making 12.

Tally Marks in Surveys

We can use tally marks while doing a survey.

For example, "What is your favourite colour?"

Ask some people what is their favourite colour.

Put a mark next to the colour they like as follows:

Yellow	////	4
Red	﷼﷼﷼	5
Blue	﷼﷼﷼ /	6
Green	/	1
Pink	////	4

When we are done, we can write the total.

Thus, we can say, 4 people liked Yellow, 5 liked Red, 6 liked Blue, only 1 liked Green and 4 people liked Pink.

The most popular colour was Blue.

Pictorial Representation of Data

Symbols, graphs and pictures are also used to represent information. Some graphs used to represent data are following.

(a) Pictograph (b) Bar graphs (or Bar charts)

Pictograph

A pictograph is a way of showing data using images. Each image stands for a certain number of things.

For example,

Here is a pictograph of how many apples were sold at the local shop over 4 months:

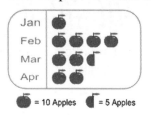

Note that each picture of an apple means 10 apples (and the half-apple picture means 5 apples).

So the pictograph is showing:

(i) In January, 10 apples were sold.

(ii) In February, 40 apples were sold.

(iii) In March, 25 apples were sold.

(iv) In April, 20 apples were sold.

It is a fun and interesting way to show data through pictograph. But it is not very accurate as in the above example we can't show just 1 apple sold, or 2 apples sold.

Bar Graph

A bar graph (also called bar chart) is a graphical display of data using bars of different heights.

We can use bar graphs to show the relative sizes of many things, such as the type of car people have, the numbers of customers a shop has on different days and so on.

Example:

A survey of 145 people revealed their favourite fruit.

Fruit	Apple	Orange	Banana	Kiwi fruit	Blueberry	Grapes
People	35	30	10	25	40	5

Draw the bar graph.

Solution:

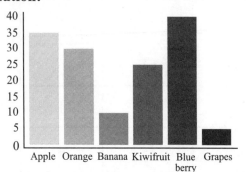

From above bar graph we can say, Blueberries are most popular and grapes are the least popular.

Pie Chart

Pie chart is a way of representing the data in a circular chart. Imagine you just did a survey to find which kind of movie your friend liked the most.

Here are the results:

Types of Movie	Comedy	Action	Romance	Drama	Science Fiction
No. of Friends	4	5	6	1	4

You could show this by pie chart as shown:

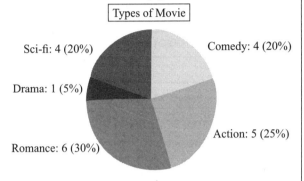

It is a really good way to show relative sizes: it is easy to see which movie types are most liked, and which are least liked, at a glance.

Notes:

(i) Read the data carefully as the smallest detail may change the meaning of the whole data collected. For example, if you are collecting data about the number of students who does not like mango, then it does not mean one do not like apple.

(ii) Record the data in tabular form because tables help to understand the data.

(iii) Try to understand the data provided carefully before jumping to answer the questions.

(iv) Relate the data given in table with charts and graphs and draw them to have better understanding of it.

(v) Be careful of the units used in tables. For example, the height of students in cm or feet.

Multiple Choice Questions

Direction (1-5): Five boats take visitors out into the sea to watch dolphins swimming. The bar chart shows the number of people that went out on each boat. Read the chart below and answer the questions that follow:

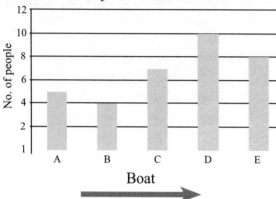

1. If Boat A: 5 :: Boat D : ?
   - (a) 4
   - (b) 5
   - (c) 10
   - (d) 8

2. Find the odd one out.
   - (a) Boat A : 5
   - (b) Boat B : 4
   - (c) Boat C : 8
   - (d) Boat E : 8

3. How many more people went to boat D than boat A?
   - (a) 5
   - (b) 4
   - (c) 3
   - (d) 2

4. How many less people went on boat C than boat E?
   - (a) 1
   - (b) 2
   - (c) 3
   - (d) 4

5. How many people went all together?
   - (a) 31
   - (b) 32
   - (c) 33
   - (d) 34

Directions (6-12): The table given below shows the number of people watching at various football grounds. Round each number to the nearest thousand and put answer in the right column. Then answer the questions that follow.

Team	No. of Players	Rounding
Aryans	2876	
Bachelors	6453	
Daredevils	3386	
Royals	4691	
Panthers	9304	
Tigers	5771	
Shera	6852	

6. Which team was watched by most people?
   - (a) Bachelors
   - (b) Tigers
   - (c) Shera
   - (d) Panthers

7. Which team was watched by least people?
   - (a) Bachelors
   - (b) Aryans
   - (c) Tigers
   - (d) Royals

8. Find the odd one out.
   - (a) Tigers
   - (b) Aryans
   - (c) Cow
   - (d) Panthers

9. How many less people watched panthers than Aryans (use rounding)?
   - (a) 4000
   - (b) 5000
   - (c) 6000
   - (d) 7000

10. How many less people watched Daredevils than Shera (use rounding)?
    - (a) 4000
    - (b) 5000
    - (c) 6000
    - (d) 7000

11. If Tigers : 6000 : : Bachelors : ?
    - (a) 5000
    - (b) 6000
    - (c) 7000
    - (d) 8000

12. If Royals : 5000 : : ? : 7000
    - (a) Bachelors
    - (b) Tigers
    - (c) Shera
    - (d) Daredevils

Direction (13-19): Golu kept a record of the birds he saw each day for five days. He presented his observation as a pictograph. Read the given pictograph and answer questions that follow.

Types of Bird	Number of Birds
Sparrow	(4 sparrows)
Seagull	(5 seagulls)
Pigeon	(8 pigeons)
Crow	(6 crows)
Parrot	(3 parrots)
Bulbul	(5 bulbuls)

1 bird is equal 10 birds.

13. How many crows did he saw?
    (a) 20   (b) 25
    (c) 30   (d) 35

14. How many more pigeons are there than sparrow?
    (a) 40   (b) 50
    (c) 30   (d) 20

15. How many fewer parrots are there than seagull?
    (a) 40   (b) 30
    (c) 20   (d) 10

16. Which bird was seen as many times as bulbul?
    (a) Sparrow   (b) Seagull
    (c) Crow   (d) Pigeon

17. State True/false for following.
    i. Pigeon was seen more than crow
    ii. Bulbul was seen less than seagull.
    iii. Sparrow was seen equal times as parrot.
    iv. Pigeon was seen more than bulbul.
    (a) FTTF   (b) TFFT
    (c) FTFT   (d) TFTF

18. Which bird was seen maximum number of times?
    (a) Bulbul   (b) Seagull
    (c) Crow   (d) Pigeon

19. Which bird was seen minimum number of times?
    (a) Parrot   (b) Crow
    (c) Bulbul   (d) Sparrow

20. Which of the following statements is/are correct?
    i. When we give information (data) about a quantity through pictures, it is called a bar graph
    ii. When we give information (data) about a quantity through horizontal or vertical bars, it is called bargraph.
    (a) Only i
    (b) Only ii
    (c) Both i and ii
    (d) Neither i nor

SECTION 2
LOGICAL REASONING

Series and Patterns

Learning Objectives:

In this chapter, students will learn about:

- Odd One Out
- Complete the Two Words
- Matching Pairs

Series

In this type of questions a series of numbers or alphabet follows a certain pattern throughout. Students are required to find out the pattern in which the series is formed.

Example: Find the missing pair of letters in the series.

FA, EC, DE, CG _____

   (a) BJ   (b) CJ

   (c) DH   (d) BI

Answer: (d)

Explanation: The answer is BI, because the pattern is to count backwards in ones for the first letter, and count forwards in two for the second letter.

First letter	F E D C B
Second letter	A C E G I

Odd One Out

These questions are designed to test candidate's ability to classify given objects on the basis of common properties.

Example: Pick the odd one out.

   (a) EHG   (b) JML

   (c) UYX   (d) TWV

Answer: (c)

Explanation: In all other groups there is a gap of one letter as in the alphabet between first and third letter.

   (a) E HG   (b) JM L

   (c) UV X   (d) TW V

Example: Identify the number which is different from the others.

   (a) 53   (b) 63

   (c) 43   (d) 83

Answer: (b)

Explanation: 53,43, 83 are prime numbers and 63 is composite a number.

Matching Pairs

These questions are designed to test the ability of a candidate to understand the relationship between two figures.

Example: Find the matching pair.

MZ is to LY as KV is to _____.

   (a) IV   (b) HV

   (c) JW   (d) GT

Answer: (c)

Explanation: MZ : LY similarly KV : JW

Example: Find the matching pair.

252 is to 5 as 343 is to _____.v

   (a) 5   (b) 4

   (c) 2   (d) 1

Answer: (b)

Explanation: 252 : 5 similarly 343 : 4

Multiple Choice Questions

1. How many circles will be there in patten 20?

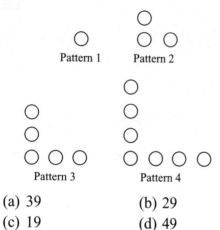

Pattern 1   Pattern 2

Pattern 3   Pattern 4

(a) 39   (b) 29
(c) 19   (d) 49

2. Which of the following figures will continue the given figure pattern?

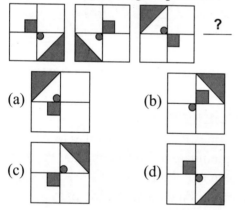

3. Which of the following figures will continue the given figure pattern?

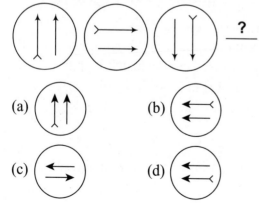

4. If the given matrix follows a certain rule row-wise or column-wise, then find the missing number.

8	4	12
10	15	1
74	?	145

(a) 112   (b) 82
(c) 14   (d) 31

5. Find the missing, if same rule is followed in all the three figures.

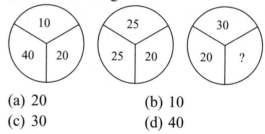

(a) 20   (b) 10
(c) 30   (d) 40

6. Which of the following options will complete the given figure _____.

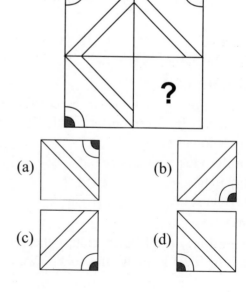

7. Which figure comes next in the given series?

(a)

(b)

(c)

(d)

8. Find the missing term in the given number series.

(a) 576   (b) 16
(c) 49   (d) 64

9. What are the next two numbers in the pattern below?
   4, 8, 16, 32, __, __
   (a) 36, 40   (b) 128, 256
   (c) 64, 128   (d) None of these

10. Find the missing numbers.

(a) 99   (b) 37
(c) 57   (d) 60

11. Find the odd one out.
    (a) DE   (b) GH
    (c) LM   (d) ON

12. Which one is different from the others?
    (a) BDC   (b) EGF
    (c) HIJ   (d) NPO

13. Identify the one that does not belong to the group.
    (a) QR   (b) NM
    (c) JI   (d) PQ

14. Which one is different from others?
    (a) 234   (b) 345
    (c) 456   (d) 657

15. Identify the one which is different from others.
    (a) 3445   (b) 4556
    (c) 7889   (d) 5567

16. Which one is different from others?
    (a) 12321   (b) 1331
    (c) 121   (d) 12341

Direction (17–26): In each of the following questions which alternative will replace the question mark.

17. FB is to GD as PM is to _____.
    (a) RO   (b) SP
    (c) RN   (d) QO

18. NA is to LF as XN is to _____.
    (a) YS   (b) VS
    (c) YM   (d) WM

19. FH is to DF as UV is to _____.
    (a) ST   (b) TX
    (c) RX   (d) TW

20. ABC is to CBA as ABCD is to _____.
    (a) ABCD   (b) BACD
    (c) CADB   (d) DCBA

21. 4 is to 16 as 16 is to _____.
    (a) 72   (b) 64
    (c) 60   (d) 33

22. 3 is to 12 as 12 is to _____.
    (a) 24   (b) 48
    (c) 36   (d) 25

23. 32 is to 16 as 16 is to _____.
    (a) 4   (b) 8
    (c) 12   (d) 47

24. 22 is to 11 as 24 is to _____.
    (a) 11   (b) 12
    (c) 14   (d) 30
25. 100 is to 50 as 90 is to _____.
    (a) 55   (b) 40
    (c) 45   (d) 85
26. Fin is to Find as Bin is to _____.
    (a) bend
    (b) bind
    (c) bond
    (d) band

Direction (27–30): Find the next letter in the series.

27. X W V U T ?
    (a) Q   (b) R   (c) S   (d) P
28. W V T Q M ?
    (a) I   (b) H   (c) G   (d) K
29. A B E J Q ?
    (a) W   (b) X   (c) Y   (d) Z
30. FX GX HY IY JZ ?
    (a) ZJ   (b) XK
    (c) JZ   (d) KZ

Coding and Decoding

> **Learning Objectives:**
> In this chapter, students will learn about:
> - Letter Coding
> - Number Coding
> - Number to Letter Coding

Coding and Decoding

a code is a 'system of signals'. Therefore, coding is a method of transmitting a message between the sender and the receiver without a third person knowing it. Decoding is a process to understand a code language.

Types of Coding

Letter Coding

In this type the alphabets in a word are replaced by certain other alphabets according to a specific rule to form its code. We are required to detect the common rule and answer the questions accordingly.

Number Coding

In this type of questions, either numerical code values are assigned to a word or alphabetical code letters are assigned to the numbers. We are required to analyse the code as per the directions.

Example: In a certain code, RIPPLE is written as 613382. How is PILLER written in that code?

    (a) 318826   (b) 318286
    (c) 618826   (d) 338816

Solution: Answer is (a).

Explanation:

The alphabets are coded as shown:

R	I	P	L	E	F
6	1	3	8	2	9

So, in PILLER,
P is coded as 3,
I as 1,
L as 8,
E as 2 and
R as 6

Thus, the code for PILLER is 318826.

Number to Letter Coding

Sometimes numbers/symbols are assigned to words.

Example: In a certain code, a number 13479 is written as AQFJL and 5268 is written as DMPN. How is 396824 written in that code?

    (a) QLPNKJ   (b) QLPNMF
    (c) QLPMNF   (d) QLPNDF

Answer (b): QLPNMF

In the given codes, the numbers are coded as shown:

1	3	4	7	9	5	2	6	8
A	Q	F	J	L	D	M	P	N

So, 396824 is coded as QLPNMF.

Example: In following questions, some capital letters (alphabet) are written in a row, their coding has been given below.

A	C	D	F	H	I	J
a	D	3	5	b	6	C

E	R	O	M	N	T	U
d	f	h	t	u	8	9

Now, find the code for 'CHATUR'

    (a) Dba89d   (b) Dba89f

    (c) D98ab1   (d) Dba98f

Answer (b)

Explanation: Observe the table and take the code for each letter so, the code for CHATUR is 'dba89f'

Example: If in a certain language, MADRAS is coded as NBESBT, how is BOMBAY coded in that language?

    (a) CPNCBX   (b) CPNCBZ

    (c) CPOCBZ   (d) CQOCBZ

Answer: (b)

Explanation: Each letter in the word is moved one step forward to obtain the corresponding letter of the code.

M + 1 => N   So,   B + 1 => C

A + 1 => B   O + 1 => P

D + 1 = >E   M + 1 => N

R + 1 => S   B + 1 => C

A + 1 => B   A+ 1 => B

S + 1 => T   Y + 1 => Z

Example: If DOWN is coded as FQYP, then how is the word WITH coded in that language?

    (a) KYJN   (b) IJYK

    (c) YKVJ   (d) JKVY

Answer: C

Explanation: The letters of the word are moved two steps forward

$$D\,O\,W\,N \xrightarrow{+2} F\,Q\,Y\,P$$

Similarly, $W\,I\,T\,H \xrightarrow{+2} Y\,K\,V\,J$

Example: If CHAIR is coded as FKDLU, then what is the code of RAID?

    (a) ULGD   (b) ULKG

    (c) ULDG   (d) UDLG

Answer: (d)

Explanation: The word is coded by moving the letters three steps forward.

$$C\,H\,A\,I\,R \xrightarrow{+3} F\,K\,D\,L\,U$$

Similarly $R\,A\,I\,D \xrightarrow{+3} U\,D\,L\,G$

Multiple Choice Questions

1. Below are given A to Z. Under each capital letter a small letter is written which is to be used as a code for the capital letter.

Letter	A	B	C	D	E	F	G	H	I	J	K	L	M
Code	e	b	n	f	Y	l	h	i	p	a	k	w	v

Letter	N	O	P	Q	R	S	T	U	V	W	X	Y	Z
Code	u	b	z	c	Q	d	o	r	s	t	j	m	G

Group of four capital letters and their equivalent codes are given below.

You have to match each group of capital letters in column I with its code in column II.

Column I	Column II
1. J D R U	(A) a e g i
2. C V F O	(B) a f q r
3. M F H B	(C) n s l b
4. J A Z H	(D) v l I x

(a) 1-B, 2-C, 3-D, 4-A
(b) 1-C, 2-B, 3-D, 4-A
(c) 1-D, 2-C, 3-A, 4-D
(d) None of these

2. If 'Red' is called 'Orange' Orange is called 'Pink' and 'Pink' is called 'Black' what is colour of apple?
(a) Red   (b) Orange
(c) Pink   (d) Black

3. If 'Red' is called 'Pencil', 'Pencil' is called 'Eraser'; 'Eraser' is called 'Notebook', What do we use to erase our mistakes on a notebook?
(a) Pencil   (b) Notebook
(c) Eraser   (d) Pen

4. If ☐ means △, △ means ⬡, ◯, ◯ means ⬠ and ⬠ means ◇, then which has no vertex?

5. If 2 means 5, 5 means 9 and 9 means 11, then which is the sum of 2 and 3?
(a) 2   (b) 5
(c) 9   (d) 11

6. If ☐ means △, △ means ☐ and ☐ means ◯, then ▱ is formed by _____.
(a) △   (b) ▭
(c) ☐   (d) ◯

7. If in a certain code, 69214 is written as HSXYR and 2387 is written as XNDU, then how will 12486 be written in the same code?
(a) ZYUDR
(b) ZYDUR
(c) YXRDH
(d) YXDRH

8. If a word is coded as 8153 and APPLE is coded as 72246, then how would you encode READ
(a) 5678   (b) 1234
(c) 4567   (d) 5673

9. If in a certain language ANSWER is coded as SNAREW, how is SQUARE written in the language?
(a) QSAUER   (b) UQSARE
(c) UQSERA   (d) ERAUQS

10. In a certain code ROPE is written as #3$% and RITE is written as #583. How is PORT written in that code?

(a) %4$#　　　　(b) $%#3

(c) $3#8　　　　(d) 583#

11. The code for same letters are shown below.

Letters	A	T	O	M	P	H	Q	S
Code	□	O	#	>	<	Δ	–	≠

Find the code for Maths.

(a) > □ O Δ #　　　　(b) < □ # Δ O

(c) – < > O □　　　　(d) □ > # < –

Direction (12–16): If MEGHA is coded as NFHIB and PEARL is coded as QFBSM, then:

12. Identify the code for VIHANG.

   (a) WJIBOI　　　　(b) WJIOBH

   (c) WIJBHO　　　　(d) WJIBOH

13. Identify the code for BHOOMI.

   (a) CIPQNI　　　　(b) CINPPJ

   (c) CIPPNJ　　　　(d) ICPPNJ

14. Identify the code for PRABHA.

   (a) QSBCIB　　　　(b) QSBCBI

   (c) QQBCIB　　　　(d) QSBCCI

15. Identify the code for AKHILESH.

   (a) BLIJMFTT　　　　(b) BLIJFMTI

   (c) BILJMFTI　　　　(d) BLIJMFTI

16. Identify the code for FAMILY.

   (a) GBNJMW　　　　(b) GBNJMZ

   (c) GBNMJVV　　　　(d) GBMWMJ

Directions (17-23): If VRUNDA is coded as XTWPFC and SWEETU is coded as UYGGVW, then:

17. Identify the code for RAKESH.

   (a) TCMGOJ　　　　(b) TCMGUJ

   (c) TCMJUG　　　　(d) TCMGUT

18. Identify the code for VARSHA.

   (a) XTCUJT　　　　(b) XCTUJC

   (c) XTCUJC　　　　(d) CTXUJC

19. Identify the code for THERMAL.

(a) VJGTOCN　　　　(b) JVGTOCN

(c) VJGOTCN　　　　(d) CTXUJC

20. Identify the code for CHINTU.

   (a) EJKPVW　　　　(b) EKJPVW

   (c) EKPVWI　　　　(d) FKLQWX

21. Identify the code for PINTU.

   (a) RKPVW　　　　(b) RKVPW

   (c) PKRVW　　　　(d) RKPWN

22. In a certain code 'TIGER' is written as 'QDFHS'. How is 'FISH' written in that code?

   (a) GERH　　　　(b) GREH

   (c) GRHE　　　　(d) GEHR

23. In a certain code 'RUAR' is written as 'URDU'. How is 'URDU' written in that code?

   (a) VXDQ　　　　(b) XUGX

   (c) ROAR　　　　(d) VZCP

24. If the letters of the word 'CYCLINDER' are arranged alphabetically, then which letter would be farthest from the first letter of word?

   (a) Y　　　　(b) N

   (c) E　　　　(d) None of these

25. If MANISH = HMSAIN, then RAMNEE = ?

   (a) AUNMEE　　　　(b) EREANM

   (c) EARMNE　　　　(d) MRAENE

26. If 'CSAT' is coded as 'EUCV', then how is 'CIVIL' written in that code?

   (a) KEXEN　　　　(b) EXKKN

   (c) EKKXN　　　　(d) EKXKN

27. If in a certain code language, 'FAVOUR' is written as '5#2@3*' and 'DANGER' is written as '6#1$7*', then how will 'FOUNDER' be written in that code language?

(a) 5@3167* (b) 521*6@2

(c) 5@7*6$2 (d) None of these

28. If 9 means 10, 10 means 15, then which is the predecessor of 1?

(a) 9 (b) 10

(c) 12 (d) 15

29. If 'X' means '÷', '÷' means '+' and '+' means '−', then which is the symbol for division?

(a) X (b) +

(c) , (d) −

Number Ranking and Alphabet Test

Learning Objectives:

In this chapter, students will learn about:

- Comparison on basis of weight, height, age, size
- Arrangement of words in Order

Number Ranking Test

In the number rankng test usually a rank puzzle is given. It may be in the form of comparison of weights, heights, ages, sizes, among the objects or persons.

Example: Ajay ranks eighteenth in a class of 49 students. What is his rank from the last?

    (a) 31   (b) 32

    (c) 19   (d) 18

Solution: Ajay's rank from the last

= (49 – 18) + 1 = 31 + 1 = 32

Study the following alphabet series to solve the example below.

A	B	C	D	E	F
N	O	P	Q	R	S

G	H	I	J	K	L	M
T	U	V	W	X	Y	Z

Example: Which letter is exactly in the middle between E and K?

    (a) G   (b) H

    (c) I   (d) J

Solution: (b)

Explanation: Write all the letters from 'E' to 'K'

    E   F   G   H   I   J   K

So, the letter in the middle of 'E' and 'K' is 'H'.

Example: Which letter is just on right side of Q?6

    (a) P   (b) O

    (c) S   (d) R

Solution: (d)

Explanation: The letter just to the right side of 'Q' means the letter which comes next to Q. i.e.'R'.

So, answer is option (d).

Example: Which letter is just on the left side of P?

    (a) O   (b) N

    (c) Q   (d) S

Solution: (a)

Explanation: The letter just on the left side of 'P' means the letter which comes before 'P', i.e. 'O'.

So, answer is option (a).

Example: Which letter is at the 9th place from the left in the alphabet series?

    (a) Q   (b) R

    (c) H   (d) I

    Answer: (d)

Explanation: 9th letter from the left means 9th letter from the first i.e.' I'.

(A B C D E F G H I J K...)

So, the answer is option d.

Example: Which letter occurs twice in PARTICULARLY, but only once in TERRIBLE?

    (a) R   (b) L

    (c) A   (d) I

Solution: (b)

Explanation: The letters A, R and L occur twice in PARTICULARLY.

The answer is L, because it appears twice in PARTICULARLY and once in TERRIBLE.

> (Not A, because there are no A's in the second word)
>
> (Not R, because there are 2 R's in the second word).

Example: Which letter is exactly between the first half of the alphabet?

    (a) F   (b) H

    (c) G   (d) I

Solution: (C)

Explanation: There are 26 letters in the English alphabet. The first half include 13 alphabets in number, i.e. from A to M.

A B C D E F G H I J K L M

The 7th letter is exactly between A and M.

7th letter is 'G'.

Alphabet Test

In the questions based on the Alphabet test, certain words are given. The candidate is required to arrange them in the order in which they are arranged in a dictionary and then to state the word which is placed in the desired place. For such questions, the candidate requires basic knowledge of the 'Dictionary Usage'. In a dictionary, the words are put in alphabetical order with respect to the second alphabet of the words and so on.

Multiple Choice Questions

1. In a row of boys, if A who is 10th from the left and B who is 9th from the right interchange their positions, A becomes 15th from the left. How many boys are there in the row?
   (a) 23　　　　　　　(b) 31
   (c) 127　　　　　　(d) 28

2. Nilu ranks 18th in a class of 49 students. What is his rank from the last?
   (a) 31　　　　　　　(b) 18
   (c) 32　　　　　　　(d) 19

3. Raju is sixth from the left end and Viru is tenth from the right end in a row of boys. If there are eight boys between Raju and Viru, how many boys are there in the row?
   (a) 24　　　　　　　(b) 26
   (c) 23　　　　　　　(d) 25

4. A class of boys stands in a single line. One boy is 19th in order from both the ends. How many boys are there in the class?
   (a) 37　　　　　　　(b) 39
   (c) 27　　　　　　　(d) 38

5. Sameer ranked 9th from the top and 38th from the bottom in a class. How many students are there in the class ?
   (a) 45　　　　　　　(b) 47
   (c) 46　　　　　　　(d) 48

6. How many 4's are there preceded by 7 but not followed by 3?
   5 9 3 2 1 7 4 2 6 9 7 4 6 1 3 2 8
   7 4 1 3 8 3 2 5 6 7 4 3 9 5 8 2 0
   1 8 7 4 6 3
   (a) Four　　　　　　(b) Three
   (c) Six　　　　　　 (d) Five

7. 517　325　639　841　792
   What will be the first digit of the second highest number after the positions of only the 2nd, 3rd digits within each number are interchanged?
   (a) 8　　　　　　　　(b) 2
   (c) 7　　　　　　　　(d) 9

8. How many numbers amongst the numbers 9 to 54 are there which are exactly divisible by 9 but not by 3 ?
   (a) 5　　　　　　　　(b) 6
   (c) 0　　　　　　　　(d) 9

9. If the positions of the first and sixth digit of the number 2796543018 are interchanged, similarly the positions of the second and seventh digits are interchanged and so on, which of the following will be on the left of the seventh digit from the left end?
   (a) 1　　　　　　　　(b) 2
   (c) 0　　　　　　　　(d) 8

10. If it is possible to form a number which is a perfect square of a two digit odd number using the second, fourth, seventh digits of the number 793142658 using each only once, which of the following is the second digit of that two-digit odd number?
    (a) 4　　　　　　　　(b) 7
    (c) 3　　　　　　　　(d) none

11. Which is the third number to the left of the number which is exactly in the middle of the following sequence of numbers?
    1 2 3 4 5 6 7 8 9 2 4 6 8 9 7 5 3
    1 9 8 7 6 5 4 3 2 1
    (a) 3　　　　　　　　(b) 5
    (c) 4　　　　　　　　(d) 7

12. In the following series of numbers, how many 1, 3, 7 have appeared together. 7 being in middle and 1, 3 on either side of?
    2 9 7 3 1 7 3 7 7 1 3 3 1 7 3 8 5
    7 1 3 7 7 1 7 3 9 0 6
    (a) 4　　　　　　　　(b) 5
    (c) 3　　　　　　　　(d) More than 5

13. If Anita is taller than Surjit but shorter than Kusum and Surjit is taller than Shubham. Who is the longest person?
    (a) Anita
    (b) Kusum
    (c) Surjit
    (d) Shubham

14. Shrikant is shorter than Nilima. Pratima is taller than Shrikant. Shubhan is taller than Nilima but shorter than Heramb. Nilima is taller than Pratima. Who will be in the middle if they stand in a row according to descending order of height?
    (a) Pratima
    (b) Shrikant
    (c) Subhash
    (d) Nilima

15. A, B, C, D and E are five rivers. A is shorter than B but longer than E. C is the longest and D is little shorter than B and little longer than A. Which is the shortest river?
    (a) B
    (b) C
    (c) D
    (d) E

16. Which letter is exactly between R and V?
    (a) S
    (b) U
    (c) T
    (d) I

17. Which letter is exactly between the English alphabet?
    (a) M
    (b) N
    (c) L
    (d) No letter

18. Which group of letters, in its number position is at interval of 6?
    (a) GMSX
    (b) IOTZ
    (c) FLRX
    (d) GKQR

19. If every alternate letter in the alphabet is deleted, then how many letter will be left in the alphabet?
    (a) 12
    (b) 13
    (c) 14
    (d) 15

20. Which letter occurs twice in INDIA and twice in BRITAIN?
    (a) T
    (b) D
    (c) I
    (d) N

21. Which letter occurs twice in SUPPORTER, but only once in OVERTAKE?
    (a) E
    (b) R
    (c) P
    (d) E

22. Which letter occurs once in GINGER, TWICE in BIGINNERR but not at all in DIVIDE?
    (a) D
    (b) N
    (c) G
    (d) E

23. In English alphabetical series, O is _____ in the series.
    (a) 5th from right end.
    (b) Between A and C
    (c) Immediate left to P
    (d) 18th From left.

24. In the English alphabetical series, D is ___ in the series.
    (a) 23rd from right
    (b) Immediate left to C
    (c) Between F and G
    (d) 3rd from left

Direction [25-28]: Study the following arrangement carefully and answer the questions given below?

    M Z R D E D 5 7 B J 1 4 N P 8 A W

25. Which of the following lies in the middle of given arrangement.
    (a) B
    (b) D
    (c) 7
    (d) W

26. Which of the following is exactly in the middle of M and E?
    (a) Z
    (b) D
    (c) R
    (d) M

27. Which of the following is third to the left of the ninth from the right end?
    (a) M
    (b) W
    (c) 8
    (d) K

28. How many English alphabets are there in this arrangement?
    - (a) 13
    - (b) 16
    - (c) 10
    - (d) 12

29. How many meaningful English words can be formed with the letters of the word 'STOP' each using only once in a word but in different sequence, starting with letter P?
    - (a) None
    - (b) Two
    - (c) One
    - (d) Three

30. How many meaningful English words can be made with the letters RBAE, using each letters only once in each word?
    - (a) None
    - (b) One
    - (c) Two
    - (d) Three

Days, Dates & Possible Combination

4

> **Learning Objectives:**
>
> In this chapter, students will learn about:
> - Days and Dates
> - Possible Combinations

1 day = 24 hours

There are 7 days in a week

Some months have 30 days and some have 31 days except February which has 28 days.

Multiple Choice Questions

1. If Tuesday falls on 4th of month, then which day will fall three days after the 24th?
   (a) Monday   (b) Tuesday
   (c) Friday   (d) Thursday

2. If the 30th January 2003 was Thursday, what was the day on 2nd March, 2003?
   (a) Sunday   (b) Thursday
   (c) Tuesday   (d) Saturday

3. If first day of the year (not a leap year) was Monday, then what was the last day of the year?
   (a) Friday   (b) Saturday
   (c) Monday   (d) Sunday

4. How many days will be there from 26th January 2008 to 15th May 2008 (both days are included)?
   (a) 111   (b) 112
   (c) 110   (d) 113

5. If the day before yesterday was Thursday, when will Sunday be?
   (a) tomorrow
   (b) today
   (c) day after tomorrow
   (d) none

6. If Day after tomorrow is Saturday, what day was 3 days before Yesterday ?
   (a) Monday   (b) Sunday
   (c) Tuesday   (d) Thursday

7. If tomorrow will be Sunday, then what was day before yesterday?
   (a) Monday   (b) Tuesday
   (c) Saturday   (d) Thursday

8. How many possible combinations of 1 apple and 1 mango can be formed from 5 apples and 5 mangoes?
   (a) 20   (b) 25
   (c) 30   (d) 35

9. If the day before yesterday was Saturday, What will be day after tomorrow?
   (a) Tuesday   (b) Wednesday
   (c) Monday   (d) Sunday

10. How many possible combinations of 1 pencil and 1 eraser from 4 pencils and 4 erasers can be formed?

   (a) 16   (b) 4

   (c) 10   (d) 15

11. Aman's birthday falls on the day just after 4th Sunday of the June 2018. The day on which Aman's birthday is _____.

June 2018						
S	M	T	W	T	F	S
					1	2

   (a) 22nd   (b) 23rd

   (c) 24th   (d) 25th

12. How many possible combinations of 1 fruit and 1 vegetable can be formed from the given table?

Fruits	Vegetables
Apple	Onion
Mango	Potato
	Brinzal

   (a) 4   (b) 2

   (c) 6   (d) None of these

13. How many possible combinations of 1 colour and 1 dress is possible to form from the given colour and dresses?

Colour	Dress
Red	Suit
Black	Saree
Yellow	Pant
	Frock
	Jeans

   (a) 15   (b) 10

   (c) 9   (d) 6

14. Rohan's birthday falls between 7th January to 11th January. Also his birthday date is an odd number. What is the date of Rohan's birthday?

   (a) 13th Jan   (b) 7th Jan

   (c) 9th Jan   (d) 10th Jan

15. Shalu's school forewell is taking place in the mid of March. What is the possible date for her school farewell?

   (a) 17th March   (b) 16th March

   (c) 15th March   (d) 18th March

16. Naina's dancing competition was held for two days before 4th Tuesday of May 20xx. The date on which Naina's dancing competition started was _____ .

May 20XX						
S	M	T	W	T	F	S
	1	2	3	4	5	6
7	8	9	10	11	12	13
14	15	16	17	18	19	20
21	22	23	24	25	26	27
28	29	30	31			

   (a) 21st May   (b) 20th May

   (c) 22nd May   (d) None of these

17. Ayaan correctly remembers that the date of his singing competition falls after 6th July and before 10th July. The friend correctly remembers that the data is even number. What will be the date of Ayaan's singing dance competition?

   (a) 9th July   (b) 6th July

   (c) 10th July   (d) 8th July

18. Tanu practices for her badminton competition on every fourth day of October 20xx starting from first Monday of the month. How many days will she practice for her badminton competition?

October 20XX						
S	M	T	W	T	F	S
	1					

(a) 7 days   (b) 8 days

(c) 10 days   (d) 11 days

19. Tarun started his project on Tuesday. He promised to his teacher that he will complete the whole project in 8 days. His work will be completed on ____.

(a) Thursday   (b) Tuesday

(c) Wednesday   (d) Sunday

20. If the given clock is 30 minutes slow, then the correct time after 20 minutes will be _____.

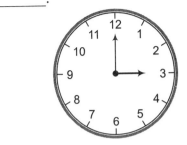

(a) 1 : 30   (b) 1 : 30

(c) 2 : 30   (d) 2 : 50

Analogy and Classification

Learning Objectives:

In this chapter, students will learn about:

- Comparison on basis of weight, height, age, size
- Arrangement of words in order

Analogy: It means similarity or bearing a resemblence.

In analogy, two pair of figures are given on either side of : : .

Classification: It means to assort items of a given group on the basis of a certain common quality they prosses.

Example: Indentify the relationship and find the missing figure.

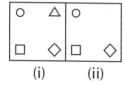 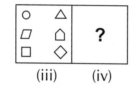

| (i) | (ii) | (iii) | (iv) |

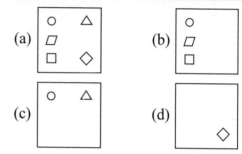

(a)   (b)

(c)   (d)

Answer: (a)

Explanation: The number of element in figure i is 4 and in figure (i) no. of elements is 3. 1 element is removed from figure (i) to get figure (ii). Similarly, same relation is used in figure (iii) to get figure (a).

Multiple Choice Questions

Directions [1-5]: There is a certain relationship between the pair of figures on the either side of :: Identify the relationship and find the missing figure.

1.
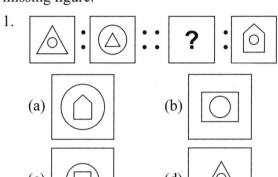

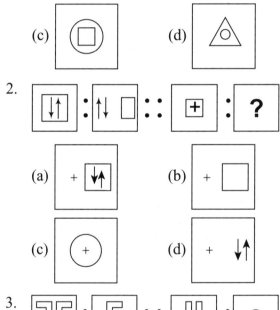

2.

3.
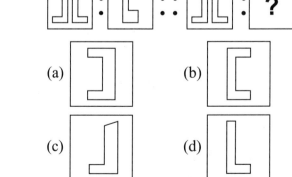

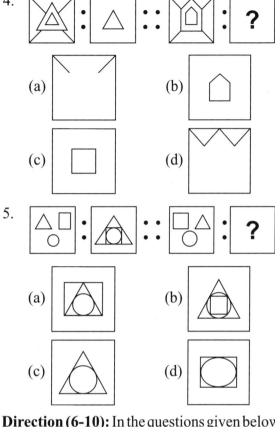

4.

5.

Direction (6-10): In the questions given below, select the word from the given alternatives.

6. 2 : 10 : : 5 : ?
   (a) 24   (b) 25
   (c) 22   (d) 21

7. Book : Library : : Fish : ?
   (a) River   (b) Sky
   (c) Flower   (d) Road

8. Weight : Kilogram : : Distance : ?
   (a) Kilogram   (b) Kilometer
   (c) Kilolitre   (d) Hours

9. CAT : TAC : : MAT : ?
   (a) MTA   (b) AMT
   (c) MAT   (d) TAM

10. Teacher : Student : : Doctor : ?
    (a) Shopkeeper   (b) Lawyer
    (c) Patient   (d) Gatekeeper

Direction (10 –15): Find the odd one out.

11. (a) Curd   (b) Butter
    (c) Cheese   (d) Oil

12. (a) 9   (b) 6
    (c) 5   (d) 3

13.
(a) 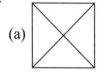   (b)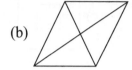

(c) 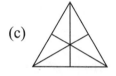   (d)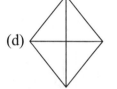

14.
(a) 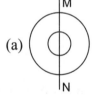   (b)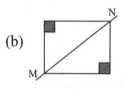

(c) 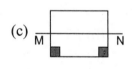   (d)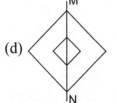

15.
(a) 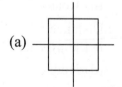   (b)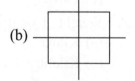

(c) 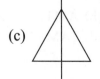   (d)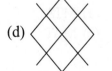

Directions (16–20): There is a relationship (i) and (ii). Select a suitable figure from the options that would replace (?) in the figure iv.

16.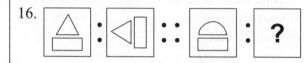

(a) 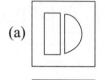   (b)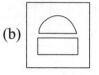

(c)    (d)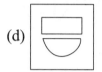

17.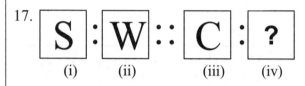
        (i)   (ii)   (iii)   (iv)

(a) B   (b) G

(c) T   (d) R

18.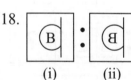
        (i)   (ii)   (iii)   (iv)

(a)    (b)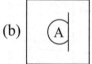

(c)    (d)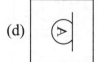

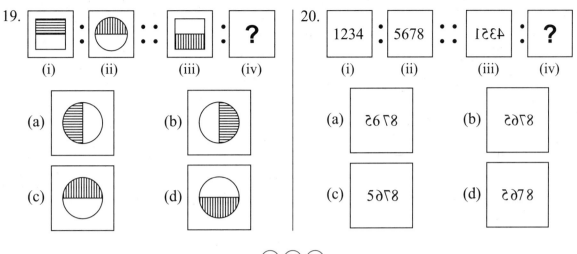

19.

(i)   (ii)   (iii)   (iv)

(a)   (b)

(c)   (d)

20.

1234 : 5678 :: ۱٤٣۱ : ?

(i)   (ii)   (iii)   (iv)

(a) ٢٦٧٨   (b) ٢٥٧٨

(c) 5٥٧٦٨   (d) ٢٥٧٨

Embedded Figures

Learning Objectives:

In this chapter, students will learn about:

- the concept of embedded figures

A figure (X) is said to be embedded in a figure (Y), if figure (Y) contains figure (X) as its part.

Example: Find the figure in which figure (X) is exactly embedded as one of its part.

 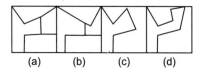

Figure (X)   (a)   (b)   (c)   (d)

Answer: (a)

Explanation:

Multiple Choice Questions

Direction (1–10): One figure is followed by four options. In one of the options, the figure similar to the problem figure is exactly embedded/concealed without any orientation. Find the option.

1.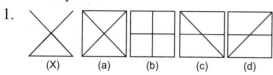
(X)   (a)   (b)   (c)   (d)

2.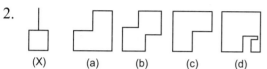
(X)   (a)   (b)   (c)   (d)

3.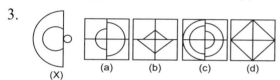
(X)   (a)   (b)   (c)   (d)

4.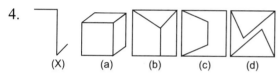
(X)   (a)   (b)   (c)   (d)

5.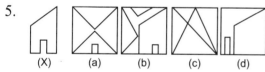
(X)   (a)   (b)   (c)   (d)

6.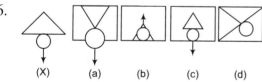
(X)   (a)   (b)   (c)   (d)

7.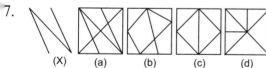
(X)   (a)   (b)   (c)   (d)

8.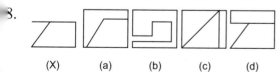
(X)   (a)   (b)   (c)   (d)

9.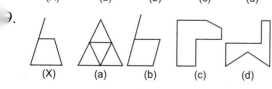
(X)   (a)   (b)   (c)   (d)

10.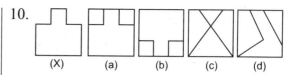
(X)   (a)   (b)   (c)   (d)

Direction (11–21): Which of the following options is exactly embedded or hidden in figure (X)?

11.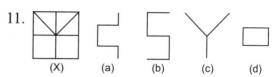
(X)   (a)   (b)   (c)   (d)

12.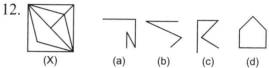
(X)   (a)   (b)   (c)   (d)

13.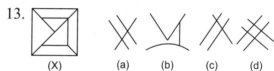
(X)   (a)   (b)   (c)   (d)

14.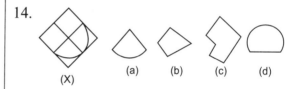
(a)   (b)   (c)   (d)
(X)

15.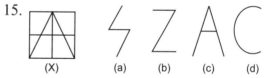
(X)   (a)   (b)   (c)   (d)

16.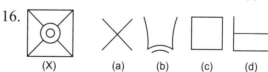
(X)   (a)   (b)   (c)   (d)

17.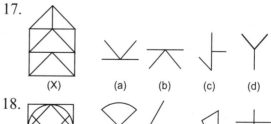
(X)   (a)   (b)   (c)   (d)

18.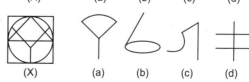
(X)   (a)   (b)   (c)   (d)

19.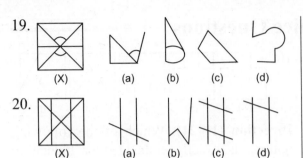

    (X)   (a)   (b)   (c)   (d)

20.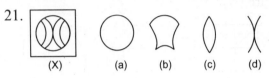

    (X)   (a)   (b)   (c)   (d)

21.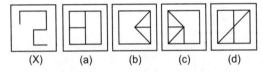

    (X)   (a)   (b)   (c)   (d)

22. In which figure from the options, figure (X) is exactly embedded as one of its part?

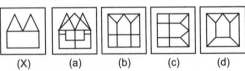

    (X)   (a)   (b)   (c)   (d)

23. Which of the answer figures in the following includes the figure X?

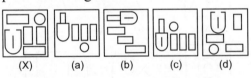

    (X)   (a)   (b)   (c)   (d)

24. Which figure includes all the specific parts of the figure 'X'?

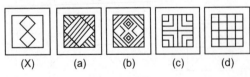

    (X)   (a)   (b)   (c)   (d)

25. Which of the following figures is exactly embedded in figure 'X'?

    (X)   (a)   (b)   (c)   (d)

26. Select a figure from the options in which figure 'X' is exactly embedded as one of its part.

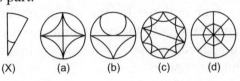

    (X)   (a)   (b)   (c)   (d)

27. In which of the following figures, the given figure 'X' is exactly embedded as one of its part?

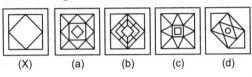

    (X)   (a)   (b)   (c)   (d)

28. In which of the following figures, the figure 'X' is included?

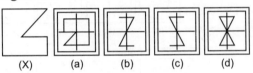

    (X)   (a)   (b)   (c)   (d)

29. Which figure from the given figures, includes the pattern of figure 'X'?

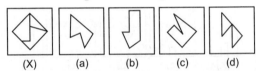

    (X)   (a)   (b)   (c)   (d)

30. Which of the following groups of alphabets is missing in the given logo?

(a) KLM   (b) OIP
(c) TKM   (d) XCD

Direction Sense Test

> **Learning Objectives:**
>
> In this chapter, students will learn about:
> - Types of directions

Direction Sense

The questions on Direction Sense are designed to test candidate's ability to sense directions.

Types of Directions

There are four main directions – East, West, North and South as shown below:

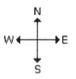

There are four cardinal directions – North-East (N-E), North-West (N-W), South-East (S-E), and South-West (S-W) as shown below:

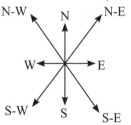

Key Points

1. At the time of sunrise if a man stands facing the east, his shadow will be towards west.

2. If a man stands facing the North, at the time of sunrise his shadow will be towards his left and at the time of sunset it will be towards his right.

3. At the time of sunset the shadow of an object is always in the east.

4. At 12:00 noon, the rays of the sun are vertically downward hence there will be no shadow.

5. Left turn → Anticlockwise direction

6. Right turn → Clockwise direction

7. Always use the diagram and table given below in case of change in direction (right or left turn).

Multiple Choice Questions

Direction (1 –10):

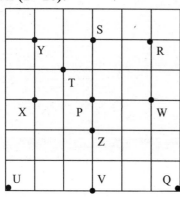

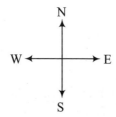

1. Which point is in the South?
   (a) X (b) Y
   (c) V (d) W

2. Which point is in the South-West?
   (a) X (b) Q
   (c) U (d) Y

3. Which point is in the East?
   (a) U (b) W
   (c) S (d) Y

4. Which point is in the West?
   (a) W (b) T
   (c) Y (d) X

5. Which point is in the North-West?
   (a) S (b) W
   (c) T (d) Z

6. Which point is in the North?
   (a) U (b) S
   (c) Q (d) V

7. Which point is in the South-east?
   (a) Q (b) S
   (c) Y (d) X

8. Which point is in the North-East?
   (a) U (b) R
   (c) W (d) X

9. Which two points are in North-West position?
   (a) T,Y (b) T,W
   (c) Y,S (d) S,R

10. Which two points are in South?
    (a) V, W (b) Z, Q
    (c) Z, T (d) Z, V

Direction (11–14): See the given figure to answer the questions.

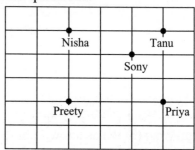

11. Who is standing to the West of Tanu?
    (a) Nisha (b) Sony
    (c) Preety (d) Priya

12. Who is standing to the East of Preety?
    (a) Nisha (b) Priya
    (c) Sony (d) Tanu

13. Who is standing to the North-east of Sony?
    (a) Nisha (b) Preety
    (c) Tanu (d) Priya

14. Who is standing to the North of Priya?
    (a) Tanu (b) Preety
    (c) Nisha (d) Sony

Direction (15–20): Use the diagram given below to answer the questions.

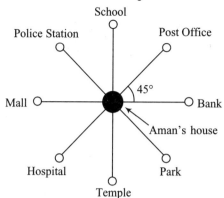

15. Aman's school is in _____ .
    (a) South
    (b) North
    (c) East
    (d) West

16. The park is in _____ .
    (a) North
    (b) South-East
    (c) East
    (d) South-West

17. Aman is facing mall. He will face _____ if he turns 45° to his left.
    (a) Temple
    (b) Police Station
    (c) Bank
    (d) Hospital

18. Aman is facing school. He will face ___ if he turns 90° to his right.
    (a) Temple
    (b) Mall
    (c) Bank
    (d) Post office

19. Aman is facing Police Station. He will face ___ if he turns 180° to his right.
    (a) Temple
    (b) Park
    (c) Mall
    (d) School

20. Aman is facing park. He will face _____ if he turns 135° to her right.
    (a) Mall
    (b) School
    (c) Park
    (d) Post-office

☺ ☺ ☺

Mirror and Water Images

Learning Objectives:

In this chapter, students will learn about:
- Mirror Images of Capital and Small Letters
- Water Images of Capital and Small Letters
- Mirror Images of Numbers
- Water Images of Numbers

Mirror Images

Reflection of an object into the mirror is called mirror image. It is obtained by inverting an object laterally.

Mirror Images of Capital Letters

Letter	Mirror-image	Letter	Mirror-image	Letter	Mirror-image
A	A	J	Ⴑᴸ	S	ꙅ
B	ꓭ	K	ꓘ	T	T
C	ꓛ	L	⅃	U	U
D	ꓷ	M	M	V	V
E	ꓱ	N	И	W	W
F	ꓞ	O	O	X	X
G	ꓜ	P	ꟼ	Y	Y
H	H	Q	Ọ	Z	Ƨ
I	I	R	Я	–	–

Mirror Images of Small Letters

Letter	Mirror-image	Letter	Mirror-image	Letter	Mirror – image
a	ɒ	j	⥾	s	ꙅ
b	d	k	ʞ	t	ɟ
c	ɔ	l	l	u	u
d	b	m	m	v	v
e	ɘ	n	ᴎ	w	w
f	ʇ	o	o	x	x
g	ǫ	p	q	y	ʏ
h	ʜ	q	p	z	ꙅ
i	i	r	ɿ		

Mirror Images of Numbers

Number	Mirror-image	Number	Mirror-image	Number	Mirror-image
1	I	4	ᔭ	7	ᓕ
2	ꙅ	5	ꙅ	8	8
3	Ɛ	6	ꓒ	9	ꟼ

Water Images

The reflection of an object, into the water, is called its water image. It is the inverted image obtained by turning the object upside down. Examples of formation of water images of some letters are given below.

Water Images of Capital Letters

Letter	A	B	C	D	E	F	G	H	I
Water Image	∀	B	C	D	E	Ⅎ	ꓚ	H	I
Letter	J	K	L	M	N	O	P	Q	R
Water Image	ꓩ	K	Ⲅ	Ⲱ	И	O	ꓭ	Ó	ʁ
Letter	S	T	U	V	W	X	Y	Z	—
Water Image	ꙅ	⊥	∩	∧	ꓟ	X	⅄	Ƨ	—

Water Images of Small Letters

Letter	a	b	c	d	e	f	g	h	i
Water Image	ɐ	ρ	ᴄ	q	ɘ	ᵴ	ᵷ	ʮ	!
Letter	j	k	l	m	n	o	p	q	r
Water Image	ꟼ	ʞ	ı	ɯ	u	o	b	d	ɹ
Letter	s	t	u	v	w	x	y	z	—
Water Image	ꙅ	ſ	ɯ	ʌ	ʍ	x	⅄	ꙅ	—

Water Images of Numbers

Letter	0	1	2	3	4	5	6	7	8	9
Water Image	0	I	ꙅ	Ɛ	ᴈ	ꙅ	ꟼ	ꓕ	8	ꟼ

Multiple Choice Questions

Direction (1–10): Choose the alternative which closely resembles the mirror image of the given combination.

1. 2 4 7 5 9 6
   (a) 6 9 5 7 4 2
   (b) �5ɘ2ⴹⴷⵦ
   (c) ⵦⴷⵦ2ɘ9
   (d) ɘ9ⵦ2ⴷⵦ

2. B R 4 A Q 1 6 H I
   (a) IH6IＱA４RB
   (b) IH6IＱA４RB
   (c) IH6IＱA４RB
   (d) IH9IＱA４ᖴᖉᗷ

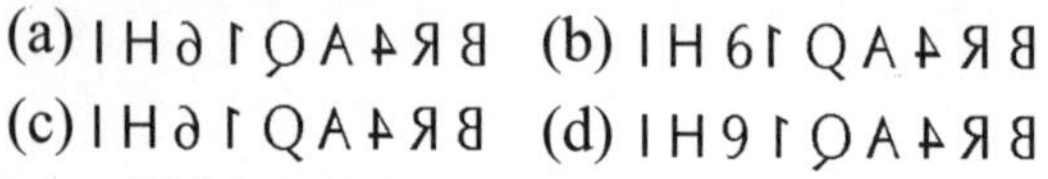

3. G E O G R A P H Y
   (a) YHᑫAᖉ⊃Oꓱꓱ
   (b) YHPARGOEG
   (c) ＾HᑫAᖉ⊃OꓱꓱY
   (d) YHᑫAᖉ⊃Oꓱꓱ

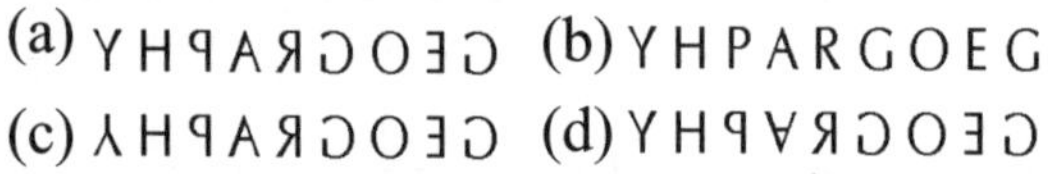

4. N A T I O N A L
   (a) ⅃AИOITAИ
   (b) ⅃AИOITAИ
   (c) ⅃AИOITAИ
   (d) LAИOITAИ

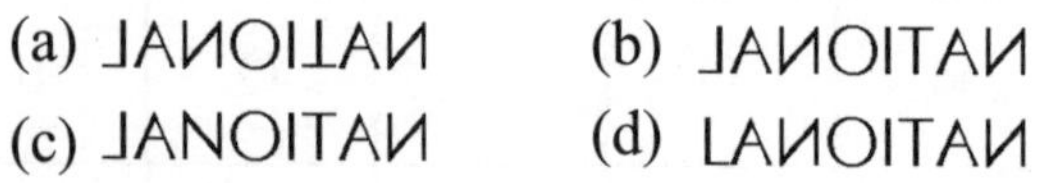

5. P A I N T E D
   (a) ꓷꓱTИIAꟼ
   (b) ꓷꓱTИIAꟼ
   (c) ꓷꓱTИIAꟼ
   (d) ꓷꓱTИIAꟼ

6. Choose the correct mirror image of the given figure (X) from amongst the four alternatives.

   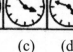
(X)   (a)   (b)   (c)   (d)

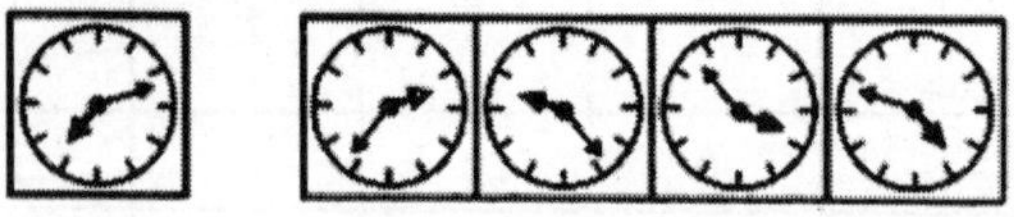

7. Choose the correct mirror image of the given figure (X) from amongst the four alternatives.

  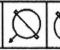
(X)   (a)   (b)   (c)   (d)

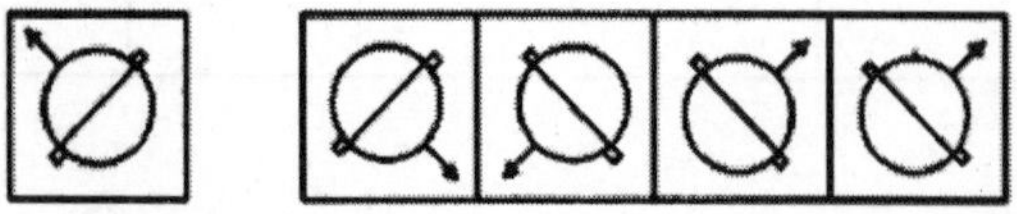

8. Choose the correct mirror image of the given figure (X) from amongst the four alternatives.

(X)   (a)   (b)   (c)   (d)

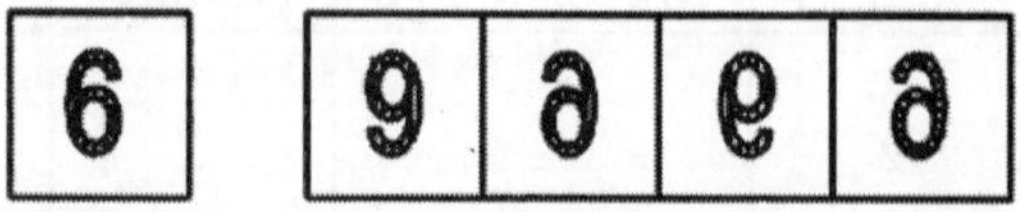

9. Choose the correct mirror image of the given figure (X) from amongst the four alternatives.

(X)   (a)   (b)   (c)   (d)

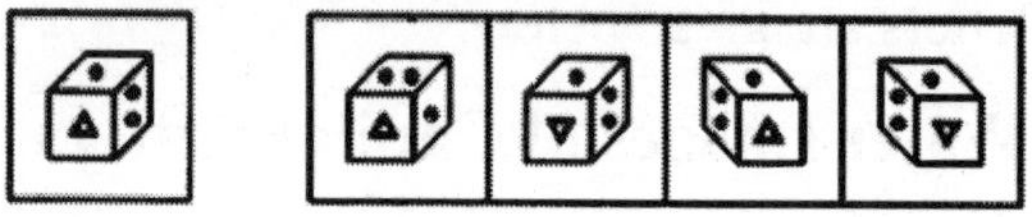

10. Choose the correct mirror image of the given figure (X) from amongst the four alternatives.

    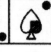
(X)   (a)   (b)   (c)   (d)

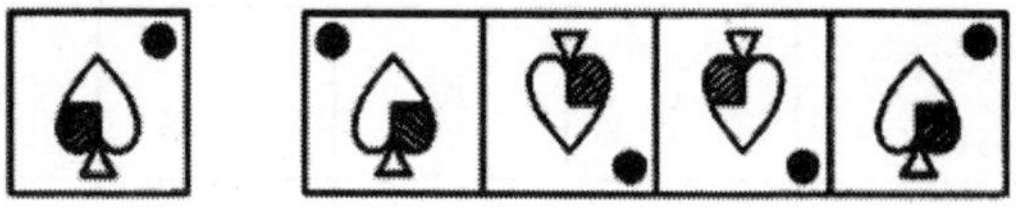

11. Choose the correct mirror image of the given figure (X) from amongst the four alternatives.

   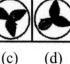
(X)   (a)   (b)   (c)   (d)

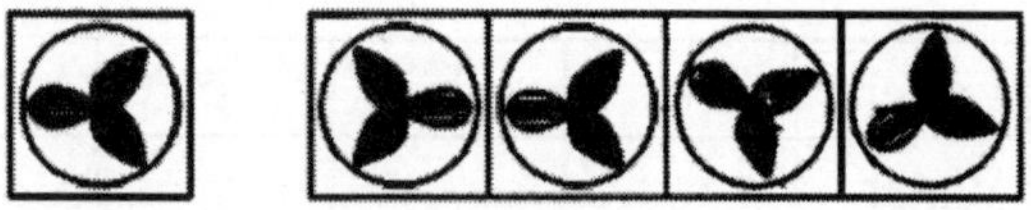

12. Choose the correct mirror image of the given figure (X) from amongst the four alternatives.

(X)   (a)   (b)   (c)   (d)

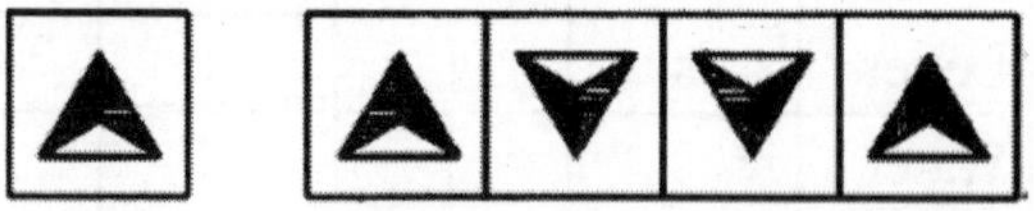

13. Choose the correct water image of the given figure (X) from amongst the four alternatives.

   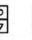
(X)   (a)   (b)   (c)   (d)

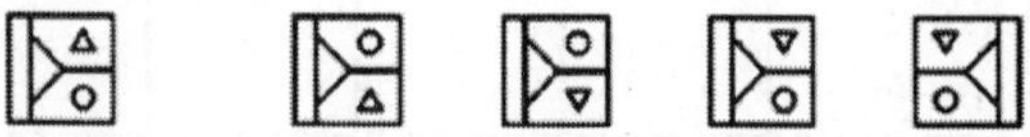

14. Choose the correct water image of the given figure (X) from amongst the four alternatives.

(X)   (a)   (b)   (c)   (d)

15. Choose the correct water image of the given figure (X) from amongst the four alternatives.

(X)   (a)   (b)   (c)   (d)

16. Choose the correct water image of the given figure (X) from amongst the four alternatives.

(X)   (a)   (b)   (c)   (d)

17. Choose the correct water image of the given figure (X) from amongst the four alternatives.

    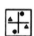   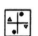

(X)   (a)   (b)   (c)   (d)

18. Choose the correct mirror image of the given figure from amongst the four alternatives.

(a)   (b)

(c)    (d)

19. Choose the alternative which closely resembles the mirror image of the given combination.

BRISK

(a) ꓘSIЯB   (b) ꓘSIЯB

(c) KSIЯB   (d) ꓘSIЯB

20. Choose the alternative which closely resembles the mirror image of the given combination.

123EBDS3FG

(a) ⅁ℲƐSᗡ8ƎƐ2Ɩ   (b) ⅁Ⅎ3Sᗡ8ƎƐ2Ɩ

(c) ⅁Ⅎ3Sᗡ8Ǝ8Ɛ2Ɩ   (d) ⅁ƐℲSᗡ8ƎƐ2Ɩ

☺☺☺

Mathematical and Analytical Reasoning

> **Learning Objectives:**
> In this chapter, students will learn about:
> - Mathematical Reasoning
> - Systematic Analysis of Information

Mathematical Reasoning

Mathematical Reasoning helps in characterizing mathematics comprehension and it also assesses logical thinking.

It helps to solve basic mathematical problems encountered in everyday life.

Example: The number of boys in a class is three times the number of girls. Which one of the following numbers cannot represent the total number of children in the class ?

(a) 48 (b) 44
(c) 42 (d) 40

Solution: c

Explanation: Let the number of girls be x then the number of boys is $3x$.

Then, total number of students $3x + x = 4x$

Hence, to find exact value of x, the total number of students must be divisible by 4.

Example: A shepherd had 17 sheep. All but nine died. How many was he left with?

(a) 17 (b) 8
(c) 9 (d) Nil

Solution: c

Explanation: 'All but nine died' means 'All except nine died' i.e. 9 sheep remained alive.

Example: In three coloured boxes – Red, Green and Blue, 108 balls are placed. There are twice as many balls in the green and red boxes combined as there are in the blue box and twice as many in the blue box as there are in the red box. How many balls are there in the green box?

(a) 18 (b) 36
(c) 45 (d) None of these

Solution: d

Explanation: Let R, G and B represent the number of balls in red, green and blue boxes, respectively.

Then,

$$R + G + B = 108 \qquad ...(i)$$
$$G + R = 2B \qquad ...(ii)$$
$$B = 2R \qquad ...(iii)$$

From (ii) and (iii), we have G + R = 2 × 2R = 4R or G = 3R.

Putting G = 3R and B = 2R in (i), we get

$$R + 3R + 2R = 108$$
$$\Rightarrow \quad 6R = 108 \Rightarrow R = 18$$

Therefore, number of balls in the green box = G = 3R = (3 × 18) = 54

Example: In a cricket match, five batsmen A, B, C, D and E scored an average of 36 runs. D scored 5 more than E; E scored 8 fewer than A; B scored as many as D and E combined;

and B and C scored 107 between them. How many runs did E score?

(a) 62   (b) 45

(c) 28   (d) 20

Solution: (d)

Explanation: Total runs scored $= (36 \times 5)$ $= 180$.

Let the runs scored by E be x.

Then, runs scored by D $= x + 5$. Runs scored by A $= x + 8$.

Runs scored by B $= x + x + 5 = 2x + 5$

Runs scored by C $= (107 - B) = 107 - (2x + 5)$ $= 102 - 2x$

So, total runs $= (x + 8) + (2x + 5) + (102 - 2x) + (x + 5) + x = 3x + 120$

Therefore, $3x + 120 = 180 \Rightarrow 3x = 60 \Rightarrow x = 20$

Example: The total number of digits used in numbering the pages of a book having 366 pages is _____.

(a) 732   (b) 990

(c) 1098   (d) 1305

Solution: (b)

Explanation: Total number of digits

$=$ (No. of digits in 1-digit page nos. + No. of digits in 2-digit page nos. + No. of digits in 3-digit page nos.)

$= (1 \times 9 + 2 \times 90 + 3 \times 267) = (9 + 180 + 801)$ $= 990$

Example: In a family, each daughter has the same number of brothers as she has sisters and each son has twice as many sisters as he has brothers. How many sons are there in the family?

(a) 2   (b) 3

(c) 4   (d) 5

Solution: (b)

Explanation: Let d and s represent the number of daughters and sons, respectively.

Then, we have:

$$d - 1 = s \text{ (i) and } 2(s - 1) = d \text{ (ii)}$$

Solving these two equations, we get: $d = 4, s = 3$.

Example: Ayush was born two years after his father's marriage. His mother is five years younger than his father but 20 years older than Ayush who is 10 years old. At what age did the father get married?

(a) 23 years   (b) 25 years

(c) 33 years   (d) 35 years

Solution: (a)

Ayush's present age = 10 years.

His mother's present age = $(10 + 20)$ years = 30 years.

Ayush's father's present age = $(30 + 5)$ years = 35 years.

Ayush's father's age at the time of Ayush's birth = $(35 - 10)$ years = 25 years.

Therefore Ayush's father's age at the time of marriage = $(25 - 2)$ years = 23 years.

Analytical Reasoning

All questions of reasoning, whether logical or numerical which require a systematic analysis of information given with question for its solution fall under this category.

Example: If day before yesterday was Saturday, what day will fall after tomorrow?

(a) Tuesday   (b) Wednesday

(c) Thursday   (d) Friday

Solution: (b)

The day before yesterday: Saturday

Yesterday : Sunday

Today : Monday

Tomorrow : Tuesday

The day after tomorrow : Wednesday

Hence, answer is option (b).

Example: Sakshi went to a movie six days ago. She goes to watch movies only on Friday. What day of the week is today?

    (a) Thursday   (b) Friday

    (c) Saturday   (d) Sunday

Solution: (a)

Six days ago : Friday

Five days ago; Saturday

Four days ago; Sunday

Three days ago; Monday

Two days ago; Tuesday

One day ago: Wednesday

Today is Thursday.

Hence, answer is option (a).

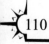

Multiple Choice Questions

1. The total of the ages of Amar, Akbar and Anthony is 80 years. What was the total of their ages three years ago?
   (a) 71 years   (b) 72 years
   (c) 74 years   (d) 77 years

2. Two bus tickets from city A to B and three tickets from city A to C cost ₹ 77 but three tickets from city A to B and two tickets from city A to C cost ₹ 73. What are the fares for cities B and C from A?
   (a) ₹ 4, ₹ 23   (b) ₹ 13, ₹ 17
   (c) ₹ 15, ₹ 14   (d) ₹ 17, ₹ 13

3. An institute organised a fete and 1/5 of the girls and 1/8 of the boys participated in the same. What fraction of the total number of students took part in the fete?
   (a) 2/13   (b) 13/40
   (c) Data inadequate   (d) None of these

4. A number of friends decided to go on a picnic and planned to spend ₹ 96 on eatables. Four of them, however, did not turn up. As a consequence, the remaining ones had to contribute ₹ 4 each extra. The number of those who attended the picnic was
   _____.
   (a) 8   (b) 12
   (c) 16   (d) 24

5. A, B, C, D and E play a game of cards. A says to B, "If you give me three cards, you will have as many as E has and if I give you three cards, you will have as many as D has." A and B together have 10 cards more than what D and E together have. If B has two cards more than what C has and the total number of cards be 133, how many cards does B have?
   (a) 22   (b) 23
   (c) 25   (d) 35

6. A pineapple costs ₹ 7 each. A watermelon costs ₹ 5 each. X spends ₹ 38 on these fruits. The number of pineapples purchased is _____.
   (a) 2
   (b) 3
   (c) 4
   (d) Data inadequate

7. A woman says, "If you reverse my own age, the figures represent my husband's age. He is, of course, senior to me and the difference between our ages is one-eleventh of their sum." The woman's age is _____.
   (a) 23 years   (b) 34 years
   (c) 45 years   (d) None of these

8. A girl counted in the following way on the fingers of her left hand: She started by calling the thumb 1, the index finger 2, middle finger 3, ring finger 4, little finger 5 and then reversed direction calling the ring finger 6, middle finger 7 and so on. She counted upto 1994. She ended counting on which finger ?
   (a) Thumb   (b) Index finger
   (c) Middle finger   (d) Ring finger

9. A man has ₹ 480 in the denomination of one-rupee notes, five-rupee notes and ten-rupee notes. The number of notes of each denomination is equal. What is the total number of notes that he has?
   (a) 45   (b) 60
   (c) 75   (d) 90

10. What is the product of all the numbers in the dial of a telephone ?
    (a) 1,58,480   (b) 1,59,450
    (c) 1,59,480   (d) None of these

11. A is 3 years older to B and 3 years younger to C, while B and D are twins. How many years older is C to D?
    (a) 2   (b) 3
    (c) 6   (d) 12

12. The 30 members of a club decided to play a badminton singles tournament. Every time a member loses a game he is out of the tournament. There are no ties. What is the minimum number of matches that must be played to determine the winner?
    (a) 15 (b) 29
    (c) 61 (d) None of these

13. In a garden, there are 10 rows and 12 columns of mango trees. The distance between the two trees is 2 metres and a distance of one metre is left from all sides of the boundary of the garden. The length of the garden is _____.
    (a) 20 m (b) 22 m
    (c) 24 m (d) 26 m

14. 12 years old Manick is three times as old as his brother Rahul. How old will Manick be when he is twice as old as Rahul?
    (a) 14 years (b) 16 years
    (c) 18 years (d) 20 years

15. A tailor had a number of shirt pieces to cut from a roll of fabric. He cut each roll of equal length into 10 pieces. He cut at the rate of 45 cuts a minute. How many rolls would be cut in 24 minutes?
    (a) 32 rolls (b) 54 rolls
    (c) 108 rolls (d) 120 rolls

16. In a class of 60 students, the number of boys and girls participating in the annual sports is in the ratio 3 : 2 respectively. The number of girls not participating in the sports is 5 more than the number of boys not participating in the sports. If the number of boys participating in the sports is 15, then how many girls are there in the class?
    (a) 20
    (b) 25
    (c) 30
    (d) Data inadequate
    (e) None of these

17. There are deer and peacocks in a zoo. By counting heads they are 80. The number of their legs is 200. How many peacocks are there?
    (a) 20 (b) 30
    (c) 50 (d) 60

18. A man wears socks of two colours – black and brown. He has altogether 20 black socks and 20 brown socks in a drawer. Supposing he has to take out the socks in the dark, how many must he take out to be sure that he has a matching pair?
    (a) 3
    (b) 20
    (c) 39
    (d) None of these

19. A motorist knows four different routes from Bristol to Birmingham. From Birmingham to Sheffield he knows three different routes and from Sheffield to Carlisle he knows two different routes. How many routes does he know from Bristol to Carlisle?
    (a) 4 (b) 8
    (c) 12 (d) 24

20. Mac has £ 3 more than Ken, but then Ken wins on the horses and trebles his money, so that he now has £ 2 more than the original amount of money that the two boys had between them. How much money did Mac and Ken have between them before Ken's win?
    (a) £ 9 (b) £ 11
    (c) £ 13 (d) £ 15

21. In a class, there are 18 boys who are over 160 cm tall. If these constitute three-fourths of the boys and the total number of boys is two-thirds of the total number of students in the class, what is the number of girls in the class?
    (a) 6 (b) 12
    (c) 18 (d) 24

22. A father is now three times as old as his son. Five years back, he was four times as old as his son. The age of the son (in years) is _____.

    (a) 12   (b) 15
    (c) 18   (d) 20

23. A waiter's salary consists of his salary and tips. During one week his tips were 5/4 of his salary. What fraction of his income came from tips?

    (a) 4/9   (b) 5/4
    (c) 5/8   (d) 5/9

24. If you write down all the numbers from 1 to 100, then how many times do you write 3?

    (a) 11   (b) 18
    (c) 20   (d) 21

25. If 100 cats kill 100 mice in 100 days, then 4 cats would kill 4 mice in how many days?

    (a) 1 day   (b) 4 days
    (c) 40 days   (d) 100 days

26. Five bells begin to toll together and toll respectively at intervals of 6, 5, 7, 10 and 12 seconds. How many times will they toll together in one hour excluding the one at the start?

    (a) 7 times   (b) 8 times
    (c) 9 times   (d) 11 times

27. A bus starts from city X. The number of women in the bus is half of the number of men. In city Y, 10 men leave the bus and five women enter. Now, number of men and women is equal. In the beginning, how many passengers entered the bus?

    (a) 15   (b) 30
    (c) 36   (d) 45

28. A, B, C, D and E play a game of cards. A says to B, "If you give me 3 cards, you will have as many as I have at this moment while if D takes 5 cards from you, he will have as many as E has." A and C together have twice as many cards as E has. B and D together also have the same number of cards as A and C taken together. If together they have 150 cards, how many cards has C got?

    (a) 28   (b) 29
    (c) 31   (d) 35

29. A farmer built a fence around his square plot. He used 27 fence poles on each side of the square. How many poles did he need altogether?

    (a) 100   (b) 104
    (c) 108   (d) None of these

30. In a city, 40% of the adults are illiterate while 85% of the children are literate. If the ratio of the adults to that of the children is 2 : 3, then what percent of the population is literate?

    (a) 20%   (b) 25%
    (c) 50%   (d) 75%

31. A is three times as old as B. C was twice-as old as A four years ago. In four years' time, A will be 31. What are the present ages of B and C?

    (a) 9 years, 46 years
    (b) 9 years, 50 years
    (c) 10 years, 46 years
    (d) 10 years, 50 years

32. Today is Varun's birthday. One year from today he will be twice as old as he was 12 years ago. How old is Varun today?

    (a) 20 years   (b) 22 years
    (c) 25 years   (d) 27 years

33. A bird shooter was asked how many birds he had in the bag. He replied that there were all sparrows but six, all pigeons but six, and all ducks but six. How many birds he had in the bag in all?
(a) 9 (b) 18
(c) 27 (d) 36

34. Mr. Johnson was to earn £ 300 and a free holiday for seven weeks' work. He worked for only 4 weeks and earned £ 30 and a free holiday. What was the value of the holiday?
(a) £ 300 (b) £ 330
(c) £ 360 (d) £ 420

35. What is the smallest number of ducks that could swim in this formation – two ducks in front of a duck, two ducks behind a duck and a duck between two ducks?
(a) 3 (b) 5
(c) 7 (d) 9

36. Three friends had dinner at a restaurant. When the bill was received, Amita paid 2/3 as much as Veena paid and Veena paid 1/2 as much as Tanya paid. What fraction of the bill did Veena pay?
(a) 1/3 (b) 3/11
(c) 12/13 (d) 5/8

37. In a class, 20% of the members own only two cars each, 40% of the remaining own three cars each and the remaining members own only one car each. Which of the following statements is definitely true from the given statements?
(a) Only 20% of the total members own three cars each.
(b) 48% of the total members own only one car each.
(c) 60% of the total members own at least two cars each.
(d) 80% of the total members own at least one car.

38. When Rahul was born, his father was 32 years older than his brother and his mother was 25 years older than his sister. If Rahul's brother is 6 years older than him and his mother is 3 years younger than his father, how old was Rahul's sister when he was born?
(a) 7 years (b) 10 years
(c) 14 years (d) 19 years

39. A certain number of horses and an equal number of men are going somewhere. Half of the owners are on their horses' back while the remaining ones are walking along leading their horses. If the number of legs walking on the ground is 70, how many horses are there?
(a) 10 (b) 12
(c) 14 (d) 16

40. Ravi's brother is 3 years senior to him. His father was 28 years of age when his sister was born while his mother was 26 years of age when he was born. If his sister was 4 years of age when his brother was born, what were the ages of Ravi's father and mother respectively when his brother was born?
(a) 32 years, 23 years
(b) 32 years, 29 years
(c) 35 years, 29 years
(d) 35 years, 33 years

☺☺☺

SECTION 3
ACHIEVERS' SECTION

Higher Order Thinking Skills (HOTS)

1. In a grazing field there are 50 goats, 40 deers and 10 children. How many legs are there in the field?
   A. 200   B. 360
   C. 380   D. 400

2. Make smallest and greatest seven-digit number and then find the difference between them.
   (a) 8999999   (b) 9999888
   (c) 8999988   (d) 8998899

3. 7 thousands, 34 hundreds and 35 ones is same as _____.
   (a) 7071   (b) 7375
   (c) 10435   (d) 7790

4. _____ thousands = 80 hundred
   (a) 8   (b) 7   (c) 6   (d) 9

5. Find the place value of 9 in the difference obtained by subtracting 70 ones from 60 hundred.
   (a) 9000   (b) 900
   (c) 90   (d) 9

6. How would you write 251 as a Roman numeral?
   (a) XCLI   (b) CXLI
   (c) CCLI   (d) XXLI

7. MMDCXXIX = _____
   (a) 2630   (b) 2590
   (c) 2629   (d) 2700

8. Which of the following statements is correct?
   (a) Symbol V, L and D can be subtracted.
   (b) Symbol X can be subtracted from L and C only
   (c) A Symbol can be repeated 4 times.
   (d) None of these

9. Find 10 less than L.
   (a) XX   (b) XL
   (c) XC   (d) XXX

10. Balance by adding roman number.

    IX + ?   XX

    (a) XI   (b) XII
    (c) X   (d) V

11. What is the sum of 1 greatest 5-digit even number and greatest 6-digit odd number?
    (a) 1099998   (b) 1099898
    (c) 1089880   (d) 1099997

12. What must be added to 4945 to get 5000?
    (a) 65   (b) 45
    (c) 55   (d) 59

13. Identify it.

    I am a 4-digit number. All my digits are different. If I add up all my digits I get 29 as sum.
    (a) 9969   (b) 5789
    (c) 4691   (c) 6789

14. Shruti had ₹22500 in the bank. She put in another ₹2550. How much more money must she put in, if she wants to have a sum of ₹40000?
    (a) ₹14500   (b) ₹14950
    (c) ₹14050   (d) ₹15050

15. When a number and 36756 both rounded off to nearest 10, we get 40000 as their sum. Find the possible number.
    (a) 3256   (b) 3245
    (c) 3242   (d) 3297

16. Find the difference of 14,235 from the sum of 13,243 + 13,243.
    (a) 11351   (b) 12251
    (c) 14531   (d) 12222

17. Select the numbers whose difference is 360.
    349   302   535   662
    (a) 535 and 302
    (b) 662 and 349
    (c) 535 and 349
    (d) 662 and 302

18. Find the difference of the place values of 9 in the following number.
    73943, 79343
    (a) 8000   (b) 8100
    (c) 7900   (d) 8900

19. Find the estimated difference by subtracting 93731 which is rounded off to nearest 1000 from 92531 which is rounded off to nearest 100.
    (a) 1700   (b) 1235
    (c) 1500   (d) 1785

20. Sara's school played thirty-two hockey matches in 2018, twenty of the matches were played at night. She attended sixteen matches out of which she played 5 night matches. How many days hockey matches did Sara miss?
    (a) 5   (b) 1
    (c) 10   (d) 2

21. If $\triangledown + \triangledown + \bigcirc = 120$ and $\bigcirc \times \bigcirc = 100$, then $\triangledown - \bigcirc = ?$
    (a) 75   (b) 25
    (c) 45   (d) 115

22. Find the value of Y to make the expression true.
    $8000 = 50 \times 80 \times Y$
    (a) 2   (b) 12
    (c) 22   (d) 10

23. Tom and Jerry sold together 120 chocolates during a sales promotion. Tom sold thrice as many chocolates than Jerry. How many chocolates did Jerry sell?
    (a) 30   (b) 40
    (c) 48   (d) 25

24. Looking at the adjoining figure, how many ancestors did Shraddha had four generations ago?

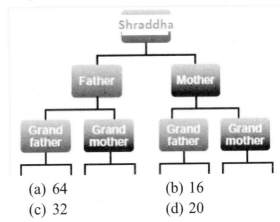

    (a) 64   (b) 16
    (c) 32   (d) 20

25. Sheetal bought 120 peaches. She found out that out of every 10 peaches, 2 are rotten and had to be thrown away. How many peaches in the end are left with her?
    (a) 90   (b) 56
    (c) 64   (d) 96

26. If product of two numbers is 100 and one of them is 10, then the other number is _____.
    (a) 4   (b) 5
    (c) 10   (d) 2

27. $65456 \div 0 =$ _____
    (a) 0   (b) 65456
    (c) 1   (d) Not defined

28. If 625 students are standing in rows and columns and there are 25 columns. Find the number of rows.
    (a) 20   (b) 15
    (c) 25   (d) 10

Higher Order Thinking Skills (HOTS)

29. I am a two-digit number. When I am divided by 9, I leave a remainder 0 and quotient 11. Who am I?
    (a) 99   (b) 11
    (c) 9   (d) None of these

30. Find the smallest number that can be added to 416 so that it can be divided by 10.
    (a) 24   (b) 14
    (c) 6   (d) 4

31. Which of the following shows all the factors of 30?
    (a) 1, 2, 3, 5, 6, 10, 15, 30
    (b) 2, 3, 5, 6, 15, 30
    (c) 1, 2, 3, 5, 6
    (d) 1, 2, 5, 6, 15, 30, 60

32. Pick the even number from the following.
    (a) 70578   (b) 734515
    (c) 93123   (d) 40321

33. What is the smallest prime factor of 55?
    (a) 55   (b) 11
    (c) 5   (d) 1

34. What is the sum of first five multiples of 5?
    (a) 65   (b) 75
    (c) 55   (d) 45

35. A number leaves ____ as remainder when divided by 2, then it is an odd number.
    (a) 2   (b) 1
    (c) 0   (d) None of these

36. Look at the given fractional shaded part.

    ■ ☐ ■ ☐ ☐ ☐ ☐ ■

    Which of the following represents the same shaded fraction?
    (a)
    (b)
    (c)
    (d)

37. Which fraction number should be placed in the box so that sum of each of them is $\dfrac{15}{7}$?

    $\dfrac{3}{7}$, $\dfrac{5}{7}$, ☐ $\dfrac{2}{7}$, $\dfrac{1}{7}$

    (a) $\dfrac{4}{7}$ (b) $\dfrac{3}{7}$
    (c) $\dfrac{5}{7}$ (d) None of these

38. The sum of two fractions is $\dfrac{9}{11}$. If one fraction is $\dfrac{1}{2}$. Find the other fraction.
    (a) $\dfrac{7}{22}$ (b) $\dfrac{9}{22}$
    (c) $\dfrac{1}{22}$ (d) $\dfrac{5}{22}$

39. Karan runs 1 km out of 4 km. Rohan runs 2 km out of 5 km and Sohan runs 3 km out of 6 km. Who runs more?
    (a) Rohan   (b) Sohan
    (c) Karan   (d) All run equally

40. What is the weight of marble P?

    (a) 300 g   (b) 250 g
    (c) 240 g   (d) 350 g

41. 4 cups of sugar of the same weight weighs 520 g. 1 glass of sugar weighs 200 g. How much heavier is 1 glass of sugar than 1 cup of sugar?
   (a) 80   (b) 50
   (c) 30   (d) 70

42. Tank A contains 3 times as much water as Tank B. How much water must be transfered from Tank A to Tank B so that each tank contains 20 litres of water?
   (a) 3 litres   (b) 20 litres
   (c) 10 litres   (d) 5 litres

43. A tailor had a piece of cloth. He cut 3 smaller pieces from cloth each $\frac{3}{4}$ m from it. If he was left with $5\frac{3}{4}$ m of cloth, then find the total length of the cloth.
   (a) 3m   (b) 6 m
   (c) 8 m   (d) 5 m

44. Sumit went to market to purchase a board game. he gave two coins of ₹5, four notes of ₹10, three notes of ₹50 and two notes of ₹500. What is the cost of board game?
   (a) ₹1500   (b) ₹1300
   (c) ₹1200   (d) ₹1000

45. Naina bought 5 chocolates. All of them were of equal price. If cost of one chocolate was ₹80 and shopkeeper gave back her ₹100, then how much money Naina gave to shopkeeper?
   (a) 500   (b) 700
   (c) 2000   (d) 1000

46.

Items	Cost per item
Pencil	₹10

Eraser	₹5
Notebook	₹20
Bottle	₹50

Look at the above table. Now find wich statement is incorrect.
   (a) Cost of 4 pencils > Cost of 1 bottle
   (b) Cost of 2 erasers = Cost of 1 pencil
   (c) Cost of 2 bottles > Cost of 2 pencils
   (d) Cost of 3 erasers < Cost of 1 notebook

47. If the cost of 1 table is equal to cost of 4 chairs, then find the cost of the table. Also, cost of 1 chair is ₹80.
   (a) ₹400   (b) ₹500
   (c) ₹320   (d) ₹450

48. How many 50 paise make 100 rupees?
   (a) 100   (b) 150
   (c) 50   (d) 200

49. Train A and Train B reach at the station at 9:00 a.m. Train A was early by 30 minutes and Train B was late by 2 hours and 30 minutes. What is the scheduled time of their arrival?
   (a) 9:30 a.m., 6:30 a.m.
   (b) 9:00 a.m., 7:00 a.m.
   (c) 10:00 a.m., 7:30 a.m.
   (d) 9:30 a.m., 7:00 a.m.

50. Sahil is going on holiday for 13 days starting from the 11th November, on what day will he come back ?
   (a) 24th November   (b) 28th November
   (c) 25th November   (d) 21st November

51. How many months are there with 31 days?
   (a) 5   (b) 10
   (c) 6   (d) 7

52. Which one is correct?

 (a) 2 hours = 720 seconds

 (b) 180 seconds = 3 minutes

 (c) 170 minutes = 2 hours 50 minutes

 (d) 2 weeks = 1170 hours

53. Sohan takes 20 minutes to walk from his home to market and then he takes 15 minutes to walk from market to his friend's house and finally from his friend's house he goes back to his house via the same path. If he leaves his house at 9:45 a.m., at what time does he reach his house?

 (a) 9:30 a.m.   (b) 10:00 a.m.

 (c) 9:55 a.m.   (d) 9:45 a.m.

54. Which of the given rectangles has the largest perimeter?

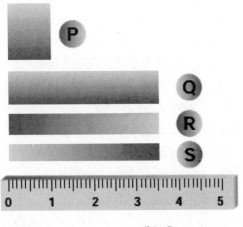

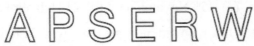

 (a) P   (b) Q

 (c) R   (d) S

55. There are _____ symmetrical alphabets and _____ non-symmetrical alphabets.

A P S E R W

 (a) 2, 4   (b) 4, 2

 (c) 5, 1   (d) 3, 3

56. If 1 ☐ is equal to 1 square unit, then find the figure with greatest perimeter.

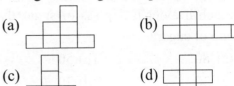

57. If side of a square is halved, then the area _____.

 (a) also get halved

 (b) becomes doubled

 (c) becomes one-fourth

 (d) remains the same

58. The given bar graph shows the height of five children. What is the difference between the height of the tallest child and the shortest child?

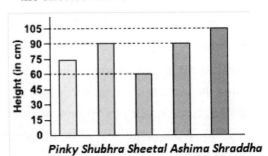

 (a) 45 cm   (b) 30 cm

 (c) 60 cm   (d) 105 cm

59. Which statement is incorrect for a bar graph?

 (a) All bars are of the same width

 (b) All bars are unevenly spaced.

 (c) Label what each bar graph represents.

 (d) Bar graphs are difficult to draw and understand.

60. Look at the given table that shows number of people who joined a comp in various years.

Year	Number of People
2013	320
2014	410
2015	205
2016	225

In which year, the number of people joined the company get halved.

(a) 2013, 2014

(b) 2014, 2015

(c) 2015, 2016

(d) 2016, 2013

Higher Order Thinking Skills (HOTS)

Model Test Paper – 1

1. Which of the given rectangles has the largest perimeter?

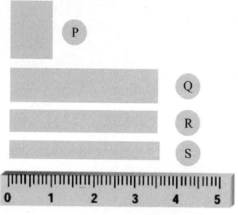

   (a) P   (b) Q
   (c) R   (d) S

2. Which one of the following has no line of symmetry?

   (a)   (b)

   (c)   (d) □

3. Find the values of P and Q respectively.

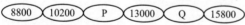

   (a) 13400, 14400   (b) 12600, 14800
   (c) 10600, 15000   (d) 11600, 14400

4. Which house has the largest value ?

   (a)   (b)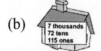

   (c)   (d)

5. 12 friends met at a party. Each friend shook hands with other exactly once. Number of handshakes took place is _____.

   (a) 66   (b) 50
   (c) 45   (d) 40

6. Riya is 17th from the front in a queue. She is 19th from the end. Then how many students are there in the queue?

   (a) 35   (b) 36
   (c) 7   (d) 20

7. Removing which of the following squares will result no change in the perimeter of the given figure?

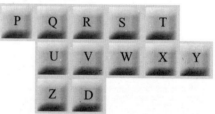

   (a) Y   (b) P
   (c) Z   (d) U

8. If there are 6 cells around one cell, 8 cells around two cells in a row, then number of cells around a row of three cells is _____.

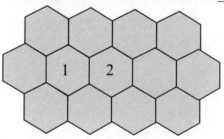

   (a) 12   (b) 10
   (c) 11   (d) 9

9. Rohan wants to move just one matchstick to make the equation correct. Which part will he take out ?

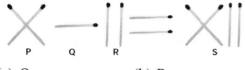

(a) Q   (b) R
(c) P   (d) S

10. Find the missing number in Fig. (X).

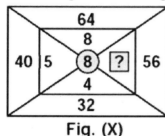

Fig. (X)

(a) 5   (b) 6
(c) 7   (d) 8

11. Which of the following is equivalent to "five lakhs one hundred and nine"?

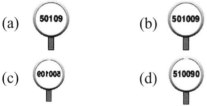

12. The given bar graph shows the height of five children. What is the difference between the height of the tallest child and the shortest child ?

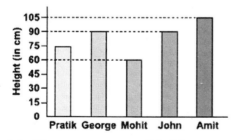

(a) 45 cm   (b) 30 cm
(c) 60 cm   (d) 105 cm

13. The perimeter of the star equals the perimeter of the hexagon (all sides are equal). If each side of the hexagon is 20 cm long, then each side of the star is _____.

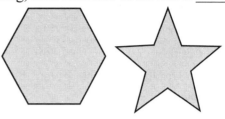

(a) 12 cm   (b) 10 cm
(c) 8 cm   (d) 9 cm

14. If $\triangledown + \triangledown + \bigcirc = 120$ and $\bigcirc \times \bigcirc = 100$, then $\triangledown - \bigcirc = ?$
(a) 15   (b) 110
(c) 45   (d) 65

15. Which of the following shows all the factors of 30?
(a) 1, 2, 3, 5, 6, 10, 15, 30
(b) 2, 3, 5, 6, 15, 30
(c) 1, 2, 3, 5, 6
(d) 1, 2, 5, 6, 15, 30, 60

16. Find the value of Y to make the expression true.
$8000 = 50 \times 80 \times Y$
(a) 2   (b) 10
(c) 20   (d) 100

17. Arrange the boxes in order, beginning from the heaviest to lightest.

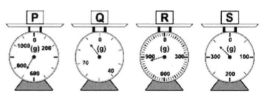

(a) P, Q, R, S
(b) Q, R, S, P
(c) R, P, S, Q
(d) S, Q, R, P

18. How much does each 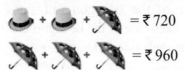 cost?

 = ₹ 720

= ₹ 960

(a) ₹ 100   (b) ₹ 320

(c) ₹ 200   (d) ₹ 240

19. Which fraction of the given figure is unshaded?

(a) 2/3   (b) 3/4   (c) 1/4   (d) 1/3

20. Where will the minute hand point after 1 hour 45 minutes from the time shown on the clock?

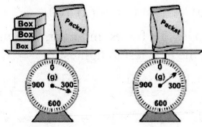

(a) 9   (b) 1   (c) 6   (d) 12

21. Roman numeral equivalent to 89 is _____.

(a) LXIL   (b) IXC

(c) XIC   (d) LXXXIX

22. What is the weight of each box?

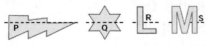

(a) 40 g   (b) 60 g

(c) 240 g   (d) 90 g

23. In which of the following dotted lines shows a line of symmetry?

(a) P   (b) Q   (c) R   (d) S

24. The product $X = 2 \times 2 \times 3 \times 5 \times 7 \times 7 \times 11 \times 13 \times 17 \times 19$ is not divisible by a number. Which is the number?

(a) 220   (b) 51

(c) 65   (d) 54

25. Find the value of X.

(a) 0   (b) 3   (c) 5   (d) 4

26. Jenny and Henry sold together 90 chocolates during a sales promotion. Henry sold twice as many chocolates than Jenny. How many chocolates did Jenny sell?

(a) 30   (b) 60

(c) 46   (d) 23

27. The capacity of a small container is 380 ml and the capacity of a big container is 1250 ml. If Aakash uses 8 small containers and 1 big container of water to fill up an empty tank, then what is the capacity of the tank?

(a) 3750 ml   (b) 4290 ml

(c) 3040 ml   (d) 4190 ml

28. Priya is practicing for a race. She uses the given map to find possible routes. The route must start from her home and end at the park. She wants to run exactly 7 km. Which of the following is the best route?

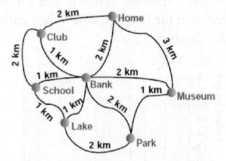

(a) Home - Bank - Museum - Park

(b) Home - Museum - Park

(c) Home - Club - School - Lake - Park

(d) Home - Bank - School - Lake - Park

29. The length of a square field is 480 m. Vishal runs 5 rounds around the field. Find the total distance run by Vishal.
    (a) 2400 m   (b) 960 m
    (c) 9600 m   (d) 4800 m

30. Looking at the adjoining figure, how many ancestors did Garima had four generations ago?

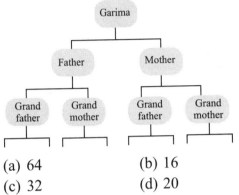

    (a) 64   (b) 16
    (c) 32   (d) 20

31. Arshan packed 726 burgers into packets of 3. He sold them at ₹ 2 per packet. How much did he get in all?
    (a) ₹ 7542   (b) ₹ 484
    (c) ₹ 242   (d) ₹ 712

32. There are 200 people in a hall. They are divided equally into 7 groups of adults and 3 groups of children. If there are 2 adults in each group, then how many children are there in each group?
    (a) 30   (b) 60
    (c) 70   (d) 62

33. Three friends, Payal, Latika and Megha are at the corners of a rectangular field. At which point should they meet so that the distances they walk to that point is minimized?

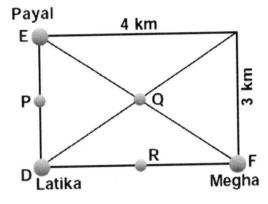

    (a) Q   (b) P
    (c) D   (d) R

34. Prerna bought 80 peaches. She found out that out of every 10 peaches, 2 are rotten and had to be thrown away. How many peaches in the end are left with her?
    (a) 70   (b) 56
    (c) 60   (d) 64

35. In a grazing field there are 60 goats, 30 deers and 10 children. How many legs are there in the field?
    (a) 200   (b) 360
    (c) 380   (d) 400

☺☺☺

Model Test Paper – 1

Model Test Paper – 2

1. How many smiling faces as shown below will there be in Pattern 10?

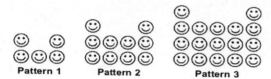

Pattern 1   Pattern 2   Pattern 3

  (a) 122   (b) 124

  (c) 126   (d) 128

2. Observe the series given below.

   1 2 2 3 3 3 4 4 4 4 5 5 5 5 5 .... What is the 20th term of the series?

   (a) 6   (b) 7

   (c) 8   (d) 5

3. Clock I shows the time when Anny starts to draw an apple.

 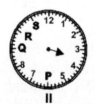

Anny takes 20 seconds to draw an apple. What will be the correct position of minute hand and second hand on clock II?

   (a) P,R   (b) P,Q

   (c) R,S   (d) Q,S

4. Weight of an apple as shown by the balance scale is _____ g.

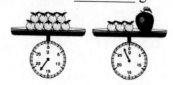

   (a) 33   (b) 22

   (c) 28   (d) 9

5. Which fraction of the following figure is shaded?

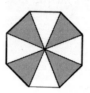

   (a) 6/8   (b) 4/8

   (c) 3/8   (d) 5/8

6. How many triangles are there in the following figure?

   (a) 29   (b) 30

   (c) 32   (d) None of these

7. Each ☐ is 1 square unit. ◺◹ are equal to ◿. Each ◺ is ½ of a square unit. Then the area of following figure is_____

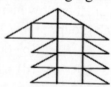

   (a) 12 sq. units   (b) 10 sq. units

   (c) 8 sq. units.   (d) 11 sq. units.

8. How many meaningful words can be formed by the letters W, N, O using all three letters? If no word is formed, then mark your answer as X and if one word is formed, mark as Y.

   (a) 2   (b) 3

   (c) Y   (d) X

9. How many meaningful words can be made from the second, third, sixth, seventh and tenth letters of the word 'MEANINGFUL', using each letter once and the words starting with Alphabet 'A'?
   (a) 0   (b) 1   (c) 2   (d) 3

10. What is the missing number?

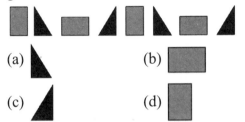

   (a) 18   (b) 19
   (c) 20   (d) 21

11. Which is the next figure in the pattern given below?

   (a)   (b)

   (c)   (d)

12. The adjoining triangle follows a number pattern.

   What are the values of P and R?
   (a) 22,8   (b) 8,32
   (c) 16,8   (d) 8,16

13. Some broken parts of mirrors are shown in the alternatives. Which one of them completes the mirror in Fig (X)?

   Fig (X)

   (a)   (b)

   (c)   (d)

14. Jiya mixed some numbers given in the adjoining box.

   Box

4	5	1	3	8	3	8	7
3	2		2	1	2	6	2
	1			4		8	9
5	2	5	3	8		9	3

   What is the fraction part of 3 among the numbers?
   (a) 5/23   (b) 4/22
   (c) 5/26   (d) 2/13

15. Rohit has a bag full of 8 red marbles, 4 blue marbles, 5 green marbles and 9 yellow marbles, all of the same size. What is the fraction of red marbles in the bag?
   (a) 8/26   (b) 4/26
   (c) 5/26   (d) 9/26

16. The diagram given below shows the pattern which Mohit uses to put tiles on his floor. Which column of tiles is missing from Mohit's floor?

   (a)   (b)

   (c)   (d)

17. Which 2 shapes should be put together to form the square in given figure?

   (a)   (b)

   (c)   (d)

18. Niti rolls a cube which has following shapes on each face.

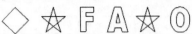

What is the fraction of symmetric shapes on the cube?
(a) 3/6　　　　　　　(b) 1/5
(c) 5/6　　　　　　　(d) 2/6

19. Sneha used a wire to make the following figure.

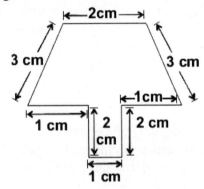

What is the length of the wire?
(a) 15 cm　　　　　　(b) 12 cm
(c) 13 cm　　　　　　(d) 14 cm

20. The length of the pencil is _____.

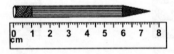

(a) 6 cm　　　　　　(b) 7 cm
(c) 7.5 cm　　　　　(d) 8 cm

21. If 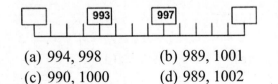 = 42, what is
⬛⬛⬛⬛?
(a) 7　　　　　　　　(b) 14
(c) 28　　　　　　　(d) 35

22. Study the number line given below. Fill the correct answer in the boxes.

| | 993 | | 997 | |

(a) 994, 998　　　　(b) 989, 1001
(c) 990, 1000　　　(d) 989, 1002

23. If ◇ × 4 = ☆, ☆ − ◇ = 330, then what is ☆ + ◇ ?
(a) 110　　　　　　　(b) 440
(c) 550　　　　　　　(d) 990

24. If the weight of the papayas is equal, then weight of 1 papaya is _____.

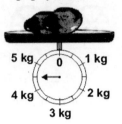

(a) $3\frac{1}{4}$ kg　　　　(b) $4\frac{1}{4}$ kg

(c) $2\frac{1}{4}$ kg　　　　(d) $1\frac{1}{4}$ kg

25. Total number of common factors of 48 and 86 is/ are ____
(a) 2　　　　　　　　(b) 3
(c) 4　　　　　　　　(d) 1

26. The standard numeral for MDCVI is ____
(a) 1606　　　　　　(b) 1305
(c) 1503　　　　　　(d) 1402

27. Arrange the sequence given below in ascending order.
1, 2, 2, 5, 4, 3, 9, 8, 7, 1, 3, 4, 5
Which of the following is the sum of middle and last digit?
(a) 13　　　　　　　(b) 12
(c) 11　　　　　　　(d) 15

28. Container B contains _____ water than container C.

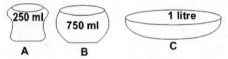

(a) 250 ml less　　　(b) 250 ml more
(c) 200 ml less　　　(d) 500 ml more

29. How will 8:25 pm written in a 24 hour clock?
    (a) 20:25 hrs   (b) 22:25 hrs
    (c) 18:25 hrs   (d) 19:25 hrs

30. What fraction of the following figures is shaded?

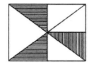

    (a) 3/4   (b) 3/5
    (c) 3/7   (d) 3/8

31. Study the addition problem given on the right.

```
    4 P 3 Q
  + R 0 6 4
  ─────────
    5 3 S 0
```

What are the values of P, Q, R, S?
    (a) 6, 0, 2, 1   (b) 2, 6, 1, 0
    (c) 2, 1, 6, 0   (d) 2, 6, 0, 1

32. 8888 = 8000 + ☐ + 8. The missing number is _____
    (a) 8   (b) 808
    (c) 88   (d) 880

33. Replace * by a number from the four alternatives.

    14/56 = 2/*
    (a) 8   (b) 26
    (c) 22   (d) 19

34. A bakery produces 780 loaves of bread in 6 days. It produces a equal number of loaves each day. How many loaves of bread does the bakery produce each day?
    (a) 130   (b) 120
    (c) 1160   (d) 1120

35. A pile of dictionary is 32 cm high. Each dictionary is 4 cm thick. How many dictionaries are there in the pile?
    (a) 8   (b) 128
    (c) 18   (d) 62

☺☺☺

Model Test Paper – 3

1. Which of the following picture cubes does the adjoining shape make?

   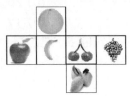

   (a)   (b)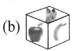

   (c)    (d)

2. Which of the following statements is false?
   (a) A rectangle is a quatridateral
   (b) A square is a rectangle
   (c) A sphere is a circle
   (d) None of these

3. When Joe got ready for school, he looked at the clock. He also saw the clock's reflection in the mirror. Which picture shows how the clock looked in the mirror?

   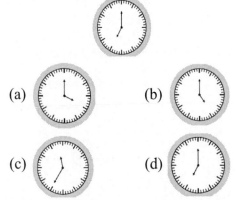

4. Priya is presently at Log Ride. She walked 5 units South and then 5 units West. Which ride did she walk to?

   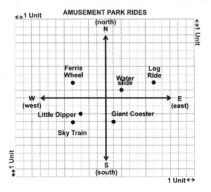

   (a) Giant Coaster
   (b) Little Dipper
   (c) Sky Train
   (d) Ferris Wheel

5. Tina and Rohit collect baseball cards. Each has the same number of cards. If Raju gives Tina and Rohit 5 more baseball cards each, who will have the greater number of baseball cards, Tina or Rohit?
   (a) Tina
   (b) Rohit
   (c) Both Tina and Rohit will have the same number of basketball cards.
   (d) There is not enough information to answer the question.

6. Which pair of numbers given in the options best completes the equation?

   $$\boxed{} \times 100 = \bigcirc$$

   (a) $\boxed{65}$ and 650
   (b) $\boxed{65}$ and $6,500$
   (c) $\boxed{605}$ and $6,500$
   (d) $\boxed{650}$ and $6,005$

7. Look at the given series:
   7, 10, 8, 11, 9, 12, _____
   What number should come next?
   (a) 7   (b) 10
   (c) 12   (d) 13

8. Tanya is older than Samrat. Mohit is older than Tanya. Samrat is older than Mohit.
   If the first two statements are true, the third statement is _____.
   (a) True   (b) False
   (c) Uncertain   (d) None of these

9. A man walks 5 km towards South and then turns to the right. After walking 3 km he turns to the left and walks 5 km. In which direction is he from the starting point?
   (a) West   (b) South
   (c) North-East   (d) South-West

10. Two positions of dice are shown below. How many points will appear opposite to the face containing 5 points?

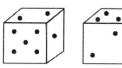

    (a) 3   (b) 1
    (c) 2   (d) 4

11. In the given figure, triangle represents 'girls', rectangle represents 'players' and circle represents 'coach'. Which part of the diagram represents girls who are players but not coach?

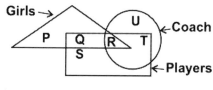

    (a) P   (b) Q
    (c) R   (d) S

12. Arrange the words given below in a meaningful sequence.
    1. Leaf   2. Fruit   3. Stem
    4. Root   5. Flower
    (a) 3,4,5,1,2   (b) 4,3,1,5,2
    (c) 4,1,3,5,2   (d) 4,3,1,2,5

13. Which number replaces the question mark?

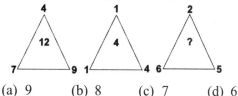

    (a) 9   (b) 8   (c) 7   (d) 6

14. Which symbol replaces the question mark?

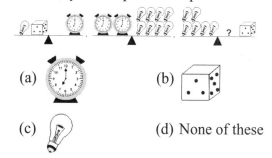

    (a)   (b)

    (c)   (d) None of these

15. Which number will replace the question mark?

5	4	7	8
6	9	5	10
3	7	2	?

    (a) 1   (b) 4
    (c) 3   (d) 6

16. What rule is used for the In-Out Machine?

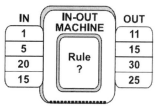

    (a) Double the number
    (b) Add 10
    (c) Add 15
    (d) Subtract 15

17. Look at Mohit's time table

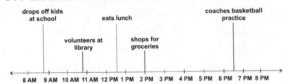

Which of the following events happens after Mohit eats lunch?

(a) Mohit volunteers at Library

(b) Mohit coaches Basketball practice

(c) Mohit drops kid at school

(d) None of these

18. Select a figure from four options which when placed in the blank space of Fig. (X) would complete the pattern.

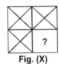

Fig. (X)

(a)
(b)
(c)
(d)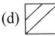

19. Kirti puts the tiles shown below into an empty bag and mixes them up.

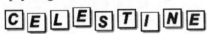

What fraction of letters are vowels?

(a) 4/10   (b) 4/9

(c) 5/9   (d) 2/9

20. The picture shows all the candy that will be placed in a machine. Each time the handle on the machine is pulled, 1 candy comes out. Alisha will pull the handle on the machine. Which color of candy is least likely to come out?

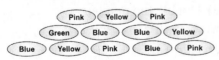

(a) Green   (b) Blue

(c) Pink   (d) Yellow

21. Which of the following represents the same value?

(a) 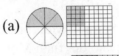   (b)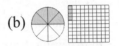

(c) 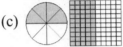   (d)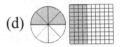

22. Which of the following figures shows only line segment PQ?

(a) P•   Q•

(b) P•————————Q•

(c) ←•P————Q•→

(d) ←•P————Q•

23. What number should go in the box to make the statement true?

$$\frac{1}{2} = \frac{\square}{8}$$

(a) 8   (b) 6

(c) 4   (d) 2

24. Which of the following is a prime number?

(a) 21   (b) 33

(c) 49   (d) 53

25. What number should go in the blank to make the given number sentence true?

$100 = 4 \times \underline{\quad} \times 5$

(a) 4   (b) 5

(c) 25   (d) 100

26. What fraction of the given figure is unshaded?

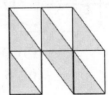

(a) 6/10　　　　(b) 3/10
(c) 5/10　　　　(d) 4/10

27. A class is making cards to give to their friends. They must use congruent (same size and shape) triangles. Look at Jamal's triangle. Jamal needs another triangle that is congruent to put on his card. Which triangle should he choose?

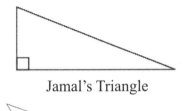

Jamal's Triangle

(a) 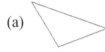　　(b)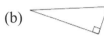

(c) 　　(d)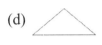

28. A number has 4 ones, 3 hundreds and 5 tens. What is the number?

(a) 354　　　　(b) 474
(c) 24315　　　(d) 31524

29. Anjali read the given pages each month. In which month did Anjali read most pages?

Pages read	
Month	Number of pages
January	4,176
February	4,416
March	4,768
April	4,716

(a) January　　　(b) February
(c) March　　　　(d) April

30. Which sign goes in the box?

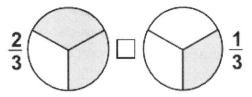

(a) <　　　　　　　(b) >
(c) =　　　　　　　(d) None of these

31. QRST is a rectangle. UVWX is a square. Find UT.

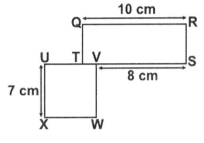

(a) 5 cm　　　　　(b) 6 cm
(c) 7 cm　　　　　(d) 8 cm

32. Which is true?
(a) 9/18 = 18/9
(b) 9 + 18 = 18 – 9
(c) 18 + 9 = 18 × 9
(d) 9 + 18 = 18 + 9

33. Tania bought these items at a sale. She went to the sale with a ₹ 500 note. How much money is left with her now?

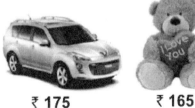

₹ 175　　　　　　₹ 165

(a) ₹ 340　　　　　(b) ₹ 260
(c) ₹ 240　　　　　(d) ₹ 160

34. Amisha and her friends decided to have a water fight on a hot summer day. They filled a bunch of water balloons and started the fight at 3:45 P.M. The water balloons lasted for 40 minutes. When all the water balloons were gone, they sprayed water with hoses for 45 minutes more, until Amisha's dad showed up with ice cream. What time was it when the water fight ended?

(a) 5:10 pm   (b) 4:25 pm
(c) 6:10 pm   (d) 5:20 pm

35. Arun works 9 hours a day. If he earns ₹ 5 an hour and works for 2 weeks everyday in the week, how much does Arun earn?

(a) ₹ 630   (b) ₹ 730
(c) ₹ 490   (d) ₹ 940

Hints and Solutions

SECTION 1: MATHEMATICAL REASONING

1. NUMBER SYSTEM

Answer Key									
1. (a)	2. (a)	3. (b)	4. (a)	5. (a)	6. (a)	7. (a)	8. (d)	9. (a)	10. (c)
11. (b)	12. (b)	13. (d)	14. (a)	15. (d)	16. (a)	17. (b)	18. (a)	19. (b)	20. (c)
21. (b)	22. (d)	23. (b)	24. (c)	25. (b)					

1. Greatest 5-digit number = 99999
2. Place value of 5 in 5,43,621
   = 5 × 100,000 = 500000
3. Smallest 6-digit number = 1,00,000
4. We have 300000 + 20000 + 4000 + 200 + 2

	L	TTh	T	H	T	O
=	3	0	0	0	0	0
	0	2	0	0	0	0
	0	0	4	0	0	0
	0	0	0	2	0	0
+	0	0	0	0	0	2
	3	2	4	2	0	2

9. We use comma to separate the periods.
13. All are 6-digit numbers except 23,456.
16. 3,44,567 has 3 lakhs.since

L	TTh	T	H	T	O
3	4	4	5	6	7

2. ROMAN NUMERALS

Answer Key									
1. (a)	2. (a)	3. (a)	4. (d)	5. (d)	6. (a)	7. (a)	8. (a)	9. (c)	10. (a)
11. (a)	12. (c)	13. (a)	14. (b)	15. (a)	16. (c)	17. (a)	18. (b)	19. (d)	20. (a)
21. (a)	22. (a)	23. (c)	24. (a)	25. (c)					

4. Here, V = 5, IV = 4, X = 10, XI = 11
    But VIIII is meaningless.
5. N is meaningless in roman numbers.
6. Roman numbers don't have symbol for zero.
9. Here CVI = 100 + 5 + 1 = 106
10. 1400 = MCD = 1000 + 500 − 100
11. We have MXVI = 1000 + 10 + 5 + 1 = 1016
12. LXXXX is meaningless.
15. We have

DCCCXXX
= 500 + 100 + 100 + 100 + 10 + 10 + 10 = 830
17. Here, 5 × 4 = VXIV
    and 5 × 4 = 20 = XX
    ∴ VXIV = XY
18. We have DVI − XXIV
    = 500 + 6 − 14 = 506 − 24
    and CDL XXX II
    = (500 − 100) + 50 + 10 + 10 + 10 + 2 = 482

3. ADDITION

Answer Key

1. (a)	2. (a)	3. (b)	4. (a)	5. (b)	6. (b)	7. (a)	8. (b)	9. (d)	10. (a)
11. (c)	12. (a)	13. (a)	14. (a)	15. (d)	16. (c)	17. (a)	18. (b)	19. (c)	20. (c)
21. (b)	22. (c)	23. (b)	24. (c)	25. (d)					

2. If we change the order of the numbers being added, the sum does not change. (Property of addition) i.e., $a + b = b + a$
4. If we add zero to any number, the sum remains the same (Property of addition)
5. If we add one to any number, the sum is always its successor.
7. We know
    addend + addend = sum
10. On adding two numbers, the result obtained is called sum.
14. 2,40,532 + 93,777 = 93,777 + 2,40,532 (Order property of addition)

22. Total distance travelled by car = Sum of 4634 and 5473

	T	H	T	O
	4	6	3	4
+	5	4	7	3
	10	1	0	7

23. Total amount = Sum of 5473 and 2335

	T	H	T	O
	5	4	7	3
+	2	3	3	5
	7	8	0	8

4. SUBTRACTION

Answer Key									
1. (b)	2. (c)	3. (a)	4. (d)	5. (a)	6. (a)	7. (c)	8. (a)	9. (a)	10. (a)
11. (a)	12. (c)	13. (b)	14. (a)	15. (a)	16. (a)	17. (a)	18. (a)	19. (c)	20. (b)
21. (a)	22. (a)	23. (a)	24. (a)	25. (a)					

2. The result after subtraction is called difference.

4. Clearly, the sum is different.

6. When we subtract a number from itself, the answer is always zero.

9. $\Box + \Box + \Box + \Box = 2400$

$4\Box = 2400$

$\Box = \dfrac{2400}{4} = 600$

$1000 - \Box = 1000 - 600 = 400 = \bigcirc$

Thus $\bigcirc = 400$

11. $1000 - ? = 900$

$? = 1000 - 900 = 10$

12. Here, $999 - 0 = 999$

and $999 - 999 = 0$

Hence both are correct.

14. Only 1 is correct.

15. $11015 + ? = 11025$

$\Rightarrow ? = 11025 - 11015 = 10$

23. Remaining eggs $= 1647 - 234 = 1413$

$$\begin{array}{r} 1647 \\ -\ 234 \\ \hline 1413 \end{array}$$

25. Required number $= 2198 - 1212$

$= 986$

$$\begin{array}{r} 2198 \\ -\ 1212 \\ \hline 0986 \end{array}$$

5. MULTIPLICATION

Answer Key									
1. (a)	2. (c)	3. (b)	4. (a)	5. (a)	6. (a)	7. (a)	8. (b)	9. (b)	10. (d)
11. (d)	12. (c)	13. (c)	14. (b)	15. (c)	16. (c)	17. (a)	18. (a)	19. (b)	20. (a)
21. (a)	22. (a)	23. (a)	24. (b)	25. (a)					

2. Multiplication is the short form of repeated addition.

3. We know $43243 \times 0 = 0$

5. We know 7074×21 and 21×7074, both are same.

7. $23 \times 100 = 2300$

10. Here $25 \times 25 = 625$

$$\begin{array}{r} 25 \\ \times\ 25 \\ \hline 125 \\ 50\times \\ \hline 625 \end{array}$$

Hints and Solutions

11. Clearly 24 is not divisible by 5 but all others are divisible by 5

12. Here 32 is odd one out.

$$11 \xrightarrow{+11} 22 \xrightarrow{+11} 33 \xrightarrow{+11} 44 \xrightarrow{+11} 55$$

∴ 32 is odd one.

21. Total no. of crayons = 79 × 93 = 7347

$$\begin{array}{r} 79 \\ \times\ 93 \\ \hline 237 \\ 711\times \\ \hline 7347 \end{array}$$

25. Rounded off 143 to nearest by 10 is 140, and rounded off 109 to nearest by 10 is 100.

Thus, 140 × 100 = 1400

This is the required product.

6. DIVISION

1. When we share equally, we divide.

2. After dividing a number, the left over is called remainder.

6. $0 \div 56 = 0$

8. If $828 \div 2 = 424$, then 424 is the quotient.

10. $0/x = 0$, where x is any number except 0.

11. $8\overline{)42}(5$

$$\begin{array}{r} \underline{40} \\ 2 \end{array}$$

Here Q = 5 and R = 2

Hence, Rahul is correct.

15. $12\overline{)7044}(587$

$$\begin{array}{r} \underline{60} \\ 104 \\ \underline{96} \\ 84 \\ \underline{84} \\ \times \end{array}$$

18. ∵ $4 \div 2 = 2$

then $40 \div 2 = 20$

$400 \div 2 = 200$

$4000 \div 2 = 2000$

20. $61\overline{)518}(8$

$$\begin{array}{r} \underline{488} \\ 30 \end{array}$$

∵ Q = 8 and R = 30

7. FACTORS AND MULTIPLES

Answer Key									
1. (a)	2. (d)	3. (d)	4. (a)	5. (d)	6. (b)	7. (b)	8. (d)	9. (b)	10. (d)
11. (a)	12. (d)	13. (a)	14. (d)	15. (c)	16. (b)	17. (a)	18. (b)	19. (d)	20. (a)
21. (b)	22. (c)	23. (a)	24. (b)	25. (c)					

1. Clearly 5 is a factor of 45 and not a multiple of 3.
3. 26, 39 and 65 are multiples of 13.
4. Clearly 48, 64 and 80 are multiples of 16 between 40 and 90.
5. Seventh multiple of $9 = 7 \times 9 = 63$
7. The given sequence is
$$2 \xrightarrow{\times 3} 6 \xrightarrow{\times 3} 18 \xrightarrow{\times 3} 54 \xrightarrow{\times 3} 162$$

10. Clearly 6 is a factor of 12.
11. 3 is not a factor of 8.
18. First 4 multiples of 3 = 3, 6, 9, 12
    First 4 multiples of 6 = 6, 12, 18, 24
    First 4 multiples of 5 = 5, 10, 15, 20
    First 4 multiples of 10 = 10, 20, 30, 40
19. Here only 5 and 25 are factors of 125.

8. FRACTIONS

Answer Key									
1. (d)	2. (d)	3. (c)	4. (a)	5. (b)	6. (b)	7. (c)	8. (a)	9. (c)	10. (c)
11. (c)	12. (a)	13. (c)	14. (a)	15. (c)	16. (d)	17. (a)	18. (a)	19. (a)	20. (c)
21. (a)	22. (a)	23. (c)	24. (c)	25. (c)					

1. $\dfrac{21}{5}$ is not a proper fraction.

2. $\dfrac{31}{8} = 3\dfrac{7}{8} = 3\left(\dfrac{7}{8}\right)$

3. $\dfrac{A}{B} = 1$ is possible when a = b

6. $\dfrac{4}{3} = 1.3$ and $\dfrac{8}{6} = 1.3$

    Hence, $\dfrac{4}{3}$ and $\dfrac{8}{6}$ are equivalent.

8. $\dfrac{2}{3}$ of an hour $= \dfrac{2}{3} \times 60$ minutes $= 40$ minutes

9. Here, $\dfrac{1}{3} + \dfrac{1}{6} + \dfrac{1}{12} = X$

    then $\dfrac{4+2+1}{12} = X \Rightarrow X = \dfrac{7}{12}$

    $\therefore \dfrac{17}{12} + X = \dfrac{17}{12} + \dfrac{7}{12} = \dfrac{24}{12} = 2$

12. We have $\dfrac{9}{15} = \dfrac{\frac{9}{3}}{\frac{15}{3}} = \dfrac{3}{5}$

13. We have $\dfrac{2}{5} \times \dfrac{3}{4} \times \dfrac{5}{8} = \dfrac{3}{16}$

22. Required no. of people $= \dfrac{20}{4} = 5$

Hints and Solutions

9. MEASUREMENT

Answer Key									
1. (c)	2. (c)	3. (d)	4. (b)	5. (d)	6. (a)	7. (b)	8. (d)	9. (b)	10. (a)
11. (b)	12. (a)	13. (c)	14. (c)	15. (d)	16. (c)	17. (b)	18. (a)	19. (c)	20. (b)

1. 2 is the tallest Giraffe.
2. Required height = 620 – 438 = 182 cm
11. Statement 3 is incorrect.
12. Here

L	mL
25	850
+ 19	390
45	240

22. We have 2550 mL = (2000 + 550) mL
$$= 2000 \text{ mL} + 550 \text{ mL}$$
$$= 2 \text{ L } 550 \text{ mL}$$
24. Required money = 4 × (4 L + 250 mL)
$$= 16 \text{ L} + 1000 \text{ mL}$$
$$= 16 \text{ L} + 1 \text{ L}$$
$$= 17 \text{ L}$$

10. MONEY

Answer Key									
1. (c)	2. (b)	3. (b)	4. (c)	5. (b)	6. (c)	7. (a)	8. (b)	9. (a)	10. (d)
11. (c)	12. (d)	13. (d)	14. (d)	15. (d)	16. (a)	17. (a)	18. (c)	19. (c)	20. (a)
21. (d)	22. (b)	23. (b)	24. (b)	25. (a)					

1. Cost of 2 pens = ₹ 24
   Cost of 1 pen = ₹ 24/2 = ₹ 12
   So, cost of 5 pens = ₹ 12 × 5 = ₹ 60
2. Sum:

	150.60
+	140.75
	291.35

   Difference:

325.50
291.35
33.15

3. Total amount Ankit needs to pay
$$= \frac{180}{2} + \frac{15}{3} = 90 + 5 = 95$$

5. Price of two chocolates $= \frac{15}{3} \times 2 = 10$
   Hence, given statement is not correct.

6. Price of one chocolate $= \frac{15}{3} = 5$

   ∴ Manpreet can buy $= \frac{122}{5}$
   $$= 24 \text{ chocolates} + 2$$

9. Total amount spent by Shraddha and Shubhra together in shopping is:
$$= (550 + 275 + 50) + (250$$
$$+ 480 + 115 + 500)$$
$$= 875 + 1345 = ₹ 2220$$

10. Amount left with Shubhra after Shopping
    = 2000 – 1345 = 655

13. Money present with Sheetal = $\dfrac{150}{2}$ = ₹ 75

22. Amount with Ashu's father
    = 10 × 50 + 5 × 80
    = 500 + 400 = 900

11. TIME AND CALENDAR

Answer Key									
1. (d)	2. (b)	3. (c)	4. (a)	5. (a)	6. (c)	7. (d)	8. (a)	9. (b)	10. (d)
11. (b)	12. (b)	13. (b)	14. (b)	15. (d)	16. (a)	17. (c)	18. (d)	19. (a)	20. (b)

1. **Month   No. of days**
   January   31
   May   31
   July   31
   November   30

2. 61 days = $\dfrac{61}{7}$ = 8 weeks + 5 days

   If today is Monday, then after 61 days
   = Monday + 5 days
   = Saturday

4. The time for 12 mid night to 12 noon is noted as am.

5. PM = Post meridian

7. 1 Year = 52 weeks + 1 day

21. Required time = 0.25 + 9.50

    = hour   min.
          9 : 50
    +   0 : 25
    _____
          9 : 75
    _____
    (60 + 15) ⇒   10 : 15

12. GEOMETRY

Answer Key									
1. (c)	2. (d)	3. (b)	4. (a)	5. (c)	6. (d)	7. (d)	8. (a)	9. (d)	10. (b)
11. (b)	12. (a)	13. (d)	14. (b)	15. (c)	16. (c)	17. (b)	18. (c)	19. (b)	20. (d)
21. (a)	22. (d)	23. (b)	24. (d)	25. (a)					

1. Six-sided polygon is called hexagon.
4. The distance between the centre and any point on the circle is called its (diameter/2) radius.

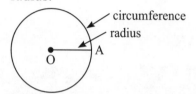

5. The perimeter of the circle is called its circumference.
14. Perimeter of square = 4 × side
    = 4 × 9 = 36 cm
16. Perimeter is measured in metre.
17. Perimeter of sheet = 2{4 + 5} = 2 × 9 = 18 m

13. PICTORIAL REPRESENTATION OF DATA

Answer Key									
1. (c)	2. (c)	3. (a)	4. (a)	5. (d)	6. (d)	7. (b)	8. (c)	9. (c)	10. (a)
11. (b)	12. (c)	13. (c)	14. (d)	15. (d)	16. (b)	17. (b)	18. (d)	19. (a)	20. (b)

1. Boat A = 5 then boat D = 10
2. Clearly Boat C : 7 Hence, C is odd one out.
3. Required people = 10 – 5 = 5
4. Required people = 8 – 7 = 1
5. Total No. of people
    = 5 + 4 + 7 + 10 + 8 = 34
20. Only statement 2 is correct.

1. SERIES AND PATTERNS

Answer Key									
1. (a)	2. (c)	3. (d)	4. (d)	5. (a)	6. (c)	7. (b)	8. (b)	9. (c)	10. (d)
11. (d)	12. (c)	13. (c)	14. (d)	15. (b)	16. (d)	17. (d)	18. (b)	19. (a)	20. (d)
21. (b)	22. (b)	23. (b)	24. (b)	25. (c)	26. (b)	27. (c)	28. (b)	29. (d)	30. (d)

12. Here $\overset{+1}{BDC}$, $\overset{+1}{EGF}$ $\overset{+1\ +1}{HIJ}$ $\overset{+1}{NPO}$

∴ HIJ is different.

17. Here $+1 \overset{F}{\underset{G}{\downarrow}} \overset{B}{\underset{D}{\downarrow}} +2$, then $+1 \overset{P}{\underset{Q}{\downarrow}} \overset{M}{\underset{O}{\downarrow}} +2$

19. Here $-2 \overset{F}{\underset{D}{\downarrow}} \overset{H}{\underset{F}{\downarrow}} -2$, then $-2 \overset{U}{\underset{S}{\downarrow}} \overset{V}{\underset{T}{\downarrow}} -2$

20. Here ABC → CBA
Then ABCD → DCBA

21. Here, $4 \to 4 \times 4 = 16$
Then $16 \to 16 \times 4 = 64$

23. Here, $32 \to \dfrac{32}{2} = 16$

Then $16 \to \dfrac{16}{2} = 8$

24. Here, $22 \to \dfrac{22}{2} = 11$

Then $24 \to \dfrac{24}{2} = 12$

25. Fin $\xrightarrow{\text{add d}}$ find
Then Bin $\xrightarrow{\text{add d}}$ Bind.

28. In the given series:
W $\xrightarrow{-0}$ V $\xrightarrow{-1}$ T $\xrightarrow{-2}$ O $\xrightarrow{-3}$ M—
So [−4] H

2. CODING AND DECODING

Answer Key									
1. (d)	2. (b)	3. (b)	4. (b)	5. (c)	6. (a)	7. (c)	8. (d)	9. (c)	10. (c)
11. (a)	12. (d)	13. (c)	14. (a)	15. (d)	16. (b)	17. (b)	18. (b)	19. (a)	20. (a)
21. (a)	22. (b)	23. (b)	24. (a)	25. (b)	26. (d)	27. (a)	28. (d)	29. (c)	

13. Given

M   E   G   H   A
+1↓ +1↓ +1↓ +1↓ +1↓
N   F   H   I   B

and   P   E   A   R   L
      +1↓ +1↓ +1↓ +1↓ +1↓
      Q   F   B   S   M

then
V   I   H   A   N   G
+1↓ +1↓ +1↓ +1↓ +1↓ +1↓
W   J   I   B   O   H

17. The code for

F   A   M   I   L   Y
+1↓ +1↓ +1↓ +1↓ +1↓ +1↓
G   B   N   J   M   Z

18.

V   R   U   N   D   A
+2↓ +2↓ +2↓ +2↓ +2↓ +2↓
X   T   W   P   F   C

and
S   W   E   E   T   U
+2↓ +2↓ +2↓ +2↓ +2↓ +2↓
U   Y   G   G   V   W

then
R   A   K   E   S   H
+2↓ +2↓ +2↓ +2↓ +2↓ +2↓
T   C   M   G   U   J

20.

T   H   E   R   M   A   L
+2↓ +2↓ +2↓ +2↓ +2↓ +2↓ +2↓
V   J   G   T   O   C   N

3. NUMBER RANKING AND ALPHABET TEST

Answer Key									
1. (a)	2. (c)	3. (a)	4. (a)	5. (c)	6. (a)	7. (c)	8. (c)	9. (b)	10. (c)
11. (c)	12. (c)	13. (c)	14. (d)	15. (d)	16. (c)	17. (d)	18. (c)	19. (b)	20. (c)
21. (b)	22. (b)	23. (c)	24. (a)	25. (a)	26. (c)	27. (d)	28. (d)	29. (b)	30. (c)

2. Nilu's ranks from the last
= (49 – 18) + 1 = 31 + 1 = 32

4. Total No. of boys in the class
= 19 + 19 – 1 = 38 – 1 = 37

7. After interchanging the 2nd and 3rd digits of all numbers. The second highest number is 329.

First digit = 7

8. Since 4 is a multiple of 3. So, there is no number between 4 and 54 which is divisible by 4 but not by 3.

11. Middle no. of this series is 4 because it is 14th no. in this series.

14. If every alternate letter in the alphabet is deleted, then total no. of letters in alphabet
= 26/2 = 13

So: third no to the left of 4 is 7

16. Letters between R and V are
R S T U V
clearly T is in middle.

17. There are 26 letters in English alphabet.
∴ No letter is exactly between the English alphabet.

20. Here I ND I A
B R I T A I N
Hence c is correct answer.

4. DAYS AND DATES AND POSSIBLE COMBINATION

					Answer Key				
1. (d)	2. (a)	3. (c)	4. (a)	5. (a)	6. (b)	7. (d)	8. (b)	9. (b)	10. (a)
11. (d)	12. (c)	13. (a)	14. (c)	15. (b)	16. (a)	17. (d)	18. (a)	19. (c)	20. (d)

7. If tomorrow will be Sunday, then today is Saturday and yesterday was Friday. Thus day before yesterday is Thursday

8. 5 Apples × 5 Mangoes = 25 possible combinations

11. 4th Sunday is on 24th June.
    Thus, just after 4th Sunday is 25th June.

12. 2 fruits × 3 vegetables = 6 possible combinations.

20. Correct time is 2 : 30
    Thus, required time is 2 : 30 + 20 minutes
    = 2 : 50

5. ANALOGY AND CLASSIFICATION

					Answer Key				
1. (a)	2. (b)	3. (d)	4. (b)	5. (a)	6. (b)	7. (a)	8. (b)	9. (d)	10. (c)
11. (d)	12. (b)	13. (c)	14. (c)	15. (c)	16. (c)	17. (c)	18. (b)	19. (d)	20. (b)

1.

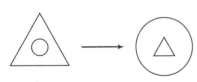

So,

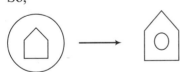

6. $2 : 2 \times 5 : : 5 : 5 \times 5$

8. Kilogram is unit of weight and Kilometre is unit of distance.

11. Oil is not a milk product.

12. 6 is even number and remaining are odd numbers.

20. i and iii are mirror images of each other.

6. EMBEDDED FIGURES

Answer Key									
1. (a)	2. (b)	3. (c)	4. (a)	5. (b)	6. (c)	7. (a)	8. (d)	9. (a)	10. (a)
11. (c)	12. (b)	13. (b)	14. (a)	15. (c)	16. (b)	17. (b)	18. (a)	19. (a)	20. (b)
21. (b)	22. (b)	23. (a)	24. (c)	25. (b)	26. (d)	27. (a)	28. (d)	29. (a)	30. (c)

1.

3.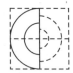

7.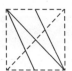

13.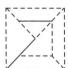

14.

20.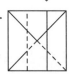

26.

7. DIRECTION SENSE TEST

Answer Key									
1. (c)	2. (c)	3. (b)	4. (d)	5. (c)	6. (b)	7. (a)	8. (b)	9. (a)	10. (d)
11. (a)	12. (b)	13. (c)	14. (a)	15. (b)	16. (b)	17. (d)	18. (c)	19. (b)	20. (a)

8. MIRROR AND WATER IMAGES

				Answer Key					
1. (d)	2. (a)	3. (a)	4. (b)	5. (b)	6. (d)	7. (c)	8. (b)	9. (c)	10. (a)
11. (a)	12. (a)	13. (b)	14. (b)	15. (c)	16. (a)	17. (c)	18. (d)	19. (a)	20. (b)

9. MATHEMATICAL AND ANALYTICAL REASONING

				Answer Key					
1. (a)	2. (b)	3. (b)	4. (b)	5. (c)	6. (c)	7. (c)	8. (b)	9. (d)	10. (d)
11. (c)	12. (b)	13. (c)	14. (b)	15. (d)	16. (c)	17. (d)	18. (a)	19. (d)	20. (c)
21. (b)	22. (b)	23. (d)	24. (c)	25. (d)	26. (b)	27. (d)	28. (a)	29. (b)	30. (d)
31. (b)	32. (c)	33. (a)	34. (b)	35. (a)	36. (b)	37. (b)	38. (b)	39. (a)	40. (a)

1. Required sum of ages = $(80 - 3 \times 3)$ years
   = $(80 - 9)$ years = 71 years

2. Let ₹ x be the fare of city B from city A and ₹ y be the fare of city C from city A.
   Then, $2x + 3y = 77$ ...(i)
   $3x + 2y = 73$ ...(ii)
   Multiplying (i) by 3 and (ii) by 2 and subtracting, we get: $5y = 85$ or $y = 17$.
   Putting $y = 17$ in (i), we get: $x = 13$.

5. According to question
   $B - 3 = E$ ...(i)
   $B + 3 = D$ ...(ii)
   $A + B = D + E + 10$ ...(iii)
   $B = C + 2$ ...(iv)
   $A + B + C + D + E = 133$ ...(v)
   From (i) and (ii), we have:
   $2B = D + E$ ...(vi)

From (iii) and (vi), we have:
$A = B + 10$ ...(vii)
Using (iv), (vi) and (vii) in (v), we get:
$(B + 10) + B + (B - 2) + 2B = 133$
$\Rightarrow 5B = 125 \Rightarrow B = 25$.

7. Let x and y be the ten's and unit's digits respectively of the numeral denoting the woman's age.
   Then, woman's age = $(10x + y)$ years; husband's age = $(10y + x)$ years.
   Therefore $(10y + x) - (10x + y)$
   $= (1/11)(10y + x + 10x + y)$
   $\Rightarrow (9y - 9x) = (1/11)(11y + 11x) = (x + y)$
   $\Rightarrow 10x = 8y \qquad \Rightarrow x = (4/5)y$
   Clearly, y should be a single-digit multiple of 5, which is 5.
   So, $x = 4$, $y = 5$.

Hence, woman's age $= 10x + y$
$= 10 \times 4 + 5 = 40 + 5 = 45$ years.

8. Clearly, while counting, the numbers associated to the thumb will be: 1, 9, 17, 25, ...
i.e. numbers of the form $(8n + 1)$.
Since $1994 = 249 \times 8 + 2$, so 1993 shall correspond to the thumb and 1994 to the index finger.

9. Let number of notes of each denomination be x.
Then, $x + 5x + 10x = 480$
$\Rightarrow 16x = 480 \quad \Rightarrow x = 30$
Hence, total number of notes
$= 3x = 3 \times 30 = 90$

10. Since one of the numbers on the dial of a telephone is zero, so the product of all the numbers on it is 0.

11. Since B and D are twins, so B = D.
Now, A = B + 3 and A = C – 3.
Thus, B + 3 = C – 3 $\Rightarrow$ D + 3 = C – 3
$\Rightarrow$ C – D = 6

12. Clearly, every member except one (i.e. the winner) must lose one game to decide the winner. Thus, minimum number of matches to be played = 30 – 1 = 29

13. Each row contains 12 plants.
There are 11 gapes between the two corner trees (11 × 2) metres and 1 metre on each side is left.
Therefore, Length = (22 + 2) m = 24 m

14. Manick's present age = 12 years, Rahul's present age = 12/3 = 4 years.
Let Manick be twice as old as Rahul after x years from now.
Then, $12 + x = 2 (4 + x)$

$\Rightarrow 12 + x = 8 + 2x \qquad \Rightarrow x = 4.$
Hence, Manick's required age
$= 12 + x = 12 + 4 = 16$ years.

15. Number of cuts made to cut a roll into 10 pieces = 9.
Therefore required number of rolls
$= (45 \times 24)/9 = 120$

16. Let the number of boys and girls participating in sports be $3x$ and $2x$ respectively.
Then, $\quad 3x = 15$ or $x = 5$
So, number of girls participating in sports
$= 2x = 2 \times 5 = 10$
Number of students not participating in sports $= 60 – (15 + 10) = 35$
Let number of boys not participating in sports be y.
Then, number of girls not participating in sports $= (35 – y)$
Therefore $(35 – y) = y + 5 \quad \Rightarrow 2y = 30$
$\Rightarrow y = 15$
So, number of girls not participating in sports $= (35 – 15) = 20$.
Hence, total number of girls in the class
$= (10 + 20) = 30$

17. Let x and y be the number of deer and peacocks in the zoo respectively. Then,
$x + y = 80$ ...(i) and
$4x + 2y = 200$ or $2x + y = 100 \qquad$ ...(ii)
Solving (i) and (ii), we get $x = 20$, $y = 60$

18. Since there are socks of only two colours, so two out of any three socks must always be of the same colour.

19. Total number of routes from Bristol to Carlisle $= (4 \times 3 \times 2) = 24$

20. Let money with Ken = x. Then, money with Mac = $x + £3$.

Now, $3x = (x + x + £3) + £2$

$\Rightarrow x = £5$

Therefore Total money with Mac and Ken = $2x + £3 = £13$

21. Let the number of boys be x. Then, $(3/4)x = 18$ or $x = 18 \times (4/3) = 24$

If total number of students is y, then $(2/3)y = 24$ or $y = 24 \times (3/2) = 36$

Therefore number of girls in the class = $(36 - 24) = 12$

22. Let son's age be x years. Then, father's age = $(3x)$ years.

Five years ago, father's age = $(3x - 5)$ years and son's age = $(x - 5)$ years.

So, $3x - 5 = 4(x - 5)$

$\Rightarrow 3x - 5 = 4x - 20 \qquad \Rightarrow x = 15$

24. Clearly, from 1 to 100, there are ten numbers with 3 as the unit's digit – 3, 13, 23, 33, 43, 53, 63, 73, 83, 93; and ten numbers with 3 as the ten's digit – 30, 31, 32, 33, 34, 35, 36, 37, 38, 39

So, required number = $10 + 10 = 20$

26. L.C.M. of 6, 5, 7, 10 and 12 is 420

So, the bells will toll together after every 420 seconds = 420/60 = 7 minutes.

Now, $7 \times 8 = 56$ and $7 \times 9 = 63$

Thus, in 1-hour (or 60 minutes), the bells will toll together 8 times, excluding the one at the start.

27. Originally, let number of women = x. Then, number of men = $2x$.

So, in city Y, we have:

$(2x - 10) = (x + 5)$ or $x = 15$

Therefore, total number of passengers in the beginning = $(x + 2x) = 3x$

$\qquad = 3 \times 15 = 45$

28. Clearly, we have:

$$A = B - 3 \qquad \text{...(i)}$$
$$D + 5 = E \qquad \text{...(ii)}$$
$$A + C = 2E \qquad \text{...(iii)}$$
$$B + D = A + C = 2E \qquad \text{...(iv)}$$
$$A + B + C + D + E = 150 \qquad \text{...(v)}$$

From (iii), (iv) and (v), we get:

$5E = 150$ or $E = 30$

Putting $E = 30$ in (ii), we get: $D = 25$

Putting $E = 30$ and $D = 25$ in (iv), we get: $B = 35$

Putting $B = 35$ in (i), we get: $A = 32$

Putting $A = 32$ and $E = 30$ in (iii), we get: $C = 28$

29. Since each pole at the corner of the plot is common to its two sides, so we have:

total number of poles needed = $27 \times 4 - 4$

$= 108 - 4 = 104$

31. We have: $A = 3B \qquad \text{...(i)}$

$C - 4 = 2(A - 4) \qquad \text{...(ii)}$

Also, $A + 4 = 31$ or $A = 31 - 4 = 27$

Putting $A = 27$ in (i), we get: $B = 9$

Putting $A = 27$ in (ii), we get $C = 50$

32. Let Varun's age today = x years.

Then, Varun's age after 1 year = $(x + 1)$ years.

Therefore $x + 1 = 2(x - 12)$

$\Rightarrow x + 1 = 2x - 24 \qquad \Rightarrow x = 25$

33. There were all sparrows but six' means that six birds were not sparrows but only pigeons and ducks. Similarly, number of sparrows + number of ducks = 6 and number of sparrows + number of pigeons = 6. This is possible when there are 3 sparrows, 3 pigeons and 3 ducks i.e. 9 birds in all.

35. Clearly, the smallest such number is 3. Three ducks can be arranged as shown above to satisfy all the three given conditions.

37. Let total number of members be 100,

    Then, number of members owning only 2 cars = 20

    Number of members owning 3 cars
    $$= 40\% \text{ of } 80 = 32$$

    Number of members owning only 1 car
    $$= 100 - (20 + 32) = 48$$

    Thus, 48% of the total members own one car each.

38. When Rahul was born, his brother's age = 6 years; his father's age = (6 + 32) years = 38 years, his mother's age = (38 − 3) years = 35 years; his sister's age = (35 − 25) years = 10 years.

39. Let number of horses = number of men = x. Then, number of legs = $4x + 2x(x/2)$ = $5x$. So, $5x = 70$ or $x = 14$

40. When Ravi's brother was born, let Ravi's father's age = x years and mother's age = y years. Then, sister's age = $(x − 28)$ years.

    So, $x − 28 = 4$ or $x = 32$

    Ravi's age = $(y − 26)$ years. age of Ravi's brother = $(y − 26 + 3)$ years = $(y − 23)$ years.

    Now, when Ravi's brother was born, his age = 0 $\Rightarrow y − 23 = 0$ or $y = 23$

SECTION3: ACHIEVERS' SECTION

HIGHER ORDER THINKING SKILLS (HOTS)

Answer Key									
1. (c)	2. (a)	3. (b)	4. (a)	5. (b)	6. (c)	7. (c)	8. (b)	9. (b)	10. (a)
11. (d)	12. (c)	13. (b)	14. (b)	15. (c)	16. (b)	17. (d)	18. (b)	19. (c)	20. (b)
21. (c)	22. (a)	23. (a)	24. (b)	25. (d)	26. (c)	27. (d)	28. (c)	29. (a)	30. (d)
31. (a)	32. (a)	33. (c)	34. (b)	35. (b)	36. (d)	37. (a)	38. (a)	39. (b)	40. (b)
41. (d)	42. (b)	43. (c)	44. (c)	45. (a)	46. (a)	47. (c)	48. (d)	49. (a)	50. (a)
51. (d)	52. (b)	53. (c)	54. (b)	55. (d)	56. (c)	57. (c)	58. (a)	59. (b)	60. (b)

MODEL TEST PAPER - 1

Answer Key									
1. (b)	2. (a)	3. (d)	4. (b)	5. (a)	6. (a)	7. (c)	8. (b)	9. (a)	10. (c)
11. (c)	12. (a)	13. (a)	14. (c)	15. (a)	16. (a)	17. (c)	18. (c)	19. (d)	20. (d)
21. (d)	22. (b)	23. (b)	24. (d)	25. (c)	26. (a)	27. (b)	28. (c)	29. (c)	30. (b)
31. (b)	32. (d)	33. (a)	34. (d)	35. (c)					

MODEL TEST PAPER - 2

Answer Key									
1. (a)	2. (a)	3. (b)	4. (d)	5. (b)	6. (d)	7. (b)	8. (b)	9. (c)	10. (b)
11. (d)	12. (b)	13. (a)	14. (c)	15. (a)	16. (a)	17. (c)	18. (c)	19. (a)	20. (c)
21. (c)	22. (b)	23. (c)	24. (c)	25. (a)	26. (a)	27. (a)	28. (d)	29. (a)	30. (c)
31. (b)	32. (d)	33. (a)	34. (a)	35. (a)					

MODEL TEST PAPER - 3

Answer Key									
1. (c)	2. (c)	3. (b)	4. (a)	5. (c)	6. (b)	7. (b)	8. (b)	9. (b)	10. (c)
11. (b)	12. (b)	13. (a)	14. (a)	15. (d)	16. (b)	17. (b)	18. (b)	19. (b)	20. (a)
21. (c)	22. (b)	23. (c)	24. (d)	25. (b)	26. (d)	27. (b)	28. (a)	29. (c)	30. (b)
31. (a)	32. (d)	33. (d)	34. (a)	35. (a)					

OMR ANSWER SHEET

1. NAME (IN ENGLISH CAPITAL LETTERS ONLY)

2. FATHER'S NAME (IN ENGLISH CAPITAL LETTERS ONLY)

Students must write and darken the respective circles completely for School Code, Class and Roll No. columns, othewise their Answer Sheets will not be evaluated.

3. SCHOOL CODE

(A) (A) (0) (0) (0) (0)
(B) (B) (1) (1) (1) (1)
(C) (C) (2) (2) (2) (2)
(D) (D) (3) (3) (3) (3)
(E) (E) (4) (4) (4) (4)
(F) (F) (5) (5) (5) (5)
(G) (G) (6) (6) (6) (6)
(H) (H) (7) (7) (7) (7)
(I) (I) (8) (8) (8) (8)
(J) (J) (9) (9) (9) (9)
(K) (K)
(L) (L)
(M) (M)
(N) (N)
(O) (O)
(P) (P)
(Q) (Q)
(R) (R)
(S) (S)
(T) (T)
(U) (U)
(V) (V)
(W) (W)
(X) (X)
(Y) (Y)
(Z) (Z)

4. % of Marks | Grade

In Last Class

Percentage	OR	Grade
(0) (0) (0)		(A)
(1) (1) (1)		(B)
(2) (2) (2)		(C)
(3) (3) (3)		(D)
(4) (4) (4)		(E)
(5) (5) (5)		(F)
(6) (6) (6)		(G)
(7) (7) (7)		(H)
(8) (8) (8)		(I)
(9) (9) (9)		(J)

5. CLASS

(0) (0)
(1) (1)
(2) (2)
(4)
(5)
(6)
(7)
(8)
(9)
(M)
(B)

6. ROLL NO.

(0) (0) (0)
(1) (1) (1)
(2) (2) (2)
(3) (3) (3)
(4) (4) (4)
(5) (5) (5)
(6) (6) (6)
(7) (7) (7)
(8) (8) (8)
(9) (9) (9)

7. GENDER

MALE ○
FEMALE ○

8. STREAM
(Only for Class XI and XII Students)

MATHEMATICS ○
BIOLOGY ○
OTHERS ○

9. MARK YOUR ANSWERS WITH HB PENCIL/BALL POINT PEN (BLUE/BLACK)

No.	A	B	C	D	No.	A	B	C	D
1.	(A)	(B)	(C)	(D)	26.	(A)	(B)	(C)	(D)
2.	(A)	(B)	(C)	(D)	27.	(A)	(B)	(C)	(D)
3.	(A)	(B)	(C)	(D)	28.	(A)	(B)	(C)	(D)
4.	(A)	(B)	(C)	(D)	29.	(A)	(B)	(C)	(D)
5.	(A)	(B)	(C)	(D)	30.	(A)	(B)	(C)	(D)
6.	(A)	(B)	(C)	(D)	31.	(A)	(B)	(C)	(D)
7.	(A)	(B)	(C)	(D)	32.	(A)	(B)	(C)	(D)
8.	(A)	(B)	(C)	(D)	33.	(A)	(B)	(C)	(D)
9.	(A)	(B)	(C)	(D)	34.	(A)	(B)	(C)	(D)
10.	(A)	(B)	(C)	(D)	35.	(A)	(B)	(C)	(D)
11.	(A)	(B)	(C)	(D)	36.	(A)	(B)	(C)	(D)
12.	(A)	(B)	(C)	(D)	37.	(A)	(B)	(C)	(D)
13.	(A)	(B)	(C)	(D)	38.	(A)	(B)	(C)	(D)
14.	(A)	(B)	(C)	(D)	39.	(A)	(B)	(C)	(D)
15.	(A)	(B)	(C)	(D)	40.	(A)	(B)	(C)	(D)
16.	(A)	(B)	(C)	(D)	41.	(A)	(B)	(C)	(D)
17.	(A)	(B)	(C)	(D)	42.	(A)	(B)	(C)	(D)
18.	(A)	(B)	(C)	(D)	43.	(A)	(B)	(C)	(D)
19.	(A)	(B)	(C)	(D)	44.	(A)	(B)	(C)	(D)
20.	(A)	(B)	(C)	(D)	45.	(A)	(B)	(C)	(D)
21.	(A)	(B)	(C)	(D)	46.	(A)	(B)	(C)	(D)
22.	(A)	(B)	(C)	(D)	47.	(A)	(B)	(C)	(D)
23.	(A)	(B)	(C)	(D)	48.	(A)	(B)	(C)	(D)
24.	(A)	(B)	(C)	(D)	49.	(A)	(B)	(C)	(D)
25.	(A)	(B)	(C)	(D)	50.	(A)	(B)	(C)	(D)

V&S Publisher, Head Office: F-2/16 Ansari Road, Daryaganj, New Delhi-110002, Ph: 011-23240026-27, Email:info@vspublishers.com
Regional Office: 5-1-707/1, Brij Bhawan (Beside Central Bank of India Lane) Bank Street, Koti, Hyderabad-500 095, Ph: 040-24737290, Email: vspublishershyd@gmail.com
Branch: Jaywant Industrial Estate, 1st Floor–108, Tardeo Road Opposite Sobo Central Mall, Mumbai - 400 034, Ph: 022-23510736, Email: vspublishersmum@gmail.com

OMR ANSWER SHEET

1. NAME (IN ENGLISH CAPITAL LETTERS ONLY)

2. FATHER'S NAME (IN ENGLISH CAPITAL LETTERS ONLY)

Students must write and darken the respective circles completely for School Code, Class and Roll No. columns, othewise their Answer Sheets will not be evaluated.

3. SCHOOL CODE

Letter columns: A B C D E F G H I J K L M N O P Q R S T U V W X Y Z (two columns)

Number columns: 0 1 2 3 4 5 6 7 8 9 (four columns)

4. % of Marks | Grade

In Last Class

Percentage OR Grade

Number columns: 0 1 2 3 4 5 6 7 8 9 (three columns)

Grade column: A B C D E F G H I J

5. CLASS

Number columns: 0 1 2 (first column) / 0 1 2 4 5 6 7 8 9 M B (second column)

6. ROLL NO.

Number columns: 0 1 2 3 4 5 6 7 8 9 (three columns)

7. GENDER

MALE ○
FEMALE ○

8. STREAM
(Only for Class XI and XII Students)

MATHEMATICS ○
BIOLOGY ○
OTHERS ○

9. MARK YOUR ANSWERS WITH HB PENCIL/BALL POINT PEN (BLUE/BLACK)

No.	Options	No.	Options
1.	Ⓐ Ⓑ Ⓒ Ⓓ	26.	Ⓐ Ⓑ Ⓒ Ⓓ
2.	Ⓐ Ⓑ Ⓒ Ⓓ	27.	Ⓐ Ⓑ Ⓒ Ⓓ
3.	Ⓐ Ⓑ Ⓒ Ⓓ	28.	Ⓐ Ⓑ Ⓒ Ⓓ
4.	Ⓐ Ⓑ Ⓒ Ⓓ	29.	Ⓐ Ⓑ Ⓒ Ⓓ
5.	Ⓐ Ⓑ Ⓒ Ⓓ	30.	Ⓐ Ⓑ Ⓒ Ⓓ
6.	Ⓐ Ⓑ Ⓒ Ⓓ	31.	Ⓐ Ⓑ Ⓒ Ⓓ
7.	Ⓐ Ⓑ Ⓒ Ⓓ	32.	Ⓐ Ⓑ Ⓒ Ⓓ
8.	Ⓐ Ⓑ Ⓒ Ⓓ	33.	Ⓐ Ⓑ Ⓒ Ⓓ
9.	Ⓐ Ⓑ Ⓒ Ⓓ	34.	Ⓐ Ⓑ Ⓒ Ⓓ
10.	Ⓐ Ⓑ Ⓒ Ⓓ	35.	Ⓐ Ⓑ Ⓒ Ⓓ
11.	Ⓐ Ⓑ Ⓒ Ⓓ	36.	Ⓐ Ⓑ Ⓒ Ⓓ
12.	Ⓐ Ⓑ Ⓒ Ⓓ	37.	Ⓐ Ⓑ Ⓒ Ⓓ
13.	Ⓐ Ⓑ Ⓒ Ⓓ	38.	Ⓐ Ⓑ Ⓒ Ⓓ
14.	Ⓐ Ⓑ Ⓒ Ⓓ	39.	Ⓐ Ⓑ Ⓒ Ⓓ
15.	Ⓐ Ⓑ Ⓒ Ⓓ	40.	Ⓐ Ⓑ Ⓒ Ⓓ
16.	Ⓐ Ⓑ Ⓒ Ⓓ	41.	Ⓐ Ⓑ Ⓒ Ⓓ
17.	Ⓐ Ⓑ Ⓒ Ⓓ	42.	Ⓐ Ⓑ Ⓒ Ⓓ
18.	Ⓐ Ⓑ Ⓒ Ⓓ	43.	Ⓐ Ⓑ Ⓒ Ⓓ
19.	Ⓐ Ⓑ Ⓒ Ⓓ	44.	Ⓐ Ⓑ Ⓒ Ⓓ
20.	Ⓐ Ⓑ Ⓒ Ⓓ	45.	Ⓐ Ⓑ Ⓒ Ⓓ
21.	Ⓐ Ⓑ Ⓒ Ⓓ	46.	Ⓐ Ⓑ Ⓒ Ⓓ
22.	Ⓐ Ⓑ Ⓒ Ⓓ	47.	Ⓐ Ⓑ Ⓒ Ⓓ
23.	Ⓐ Ⓑ Ⓒ Ⓓ	48.	Ⓐ Ⓑ Ⓒ Ⓓ
24.	Ⓐ Ⓑ Ⓒ Ⓓ	49.	Ⓐ Ⓑ Ⓒ Ⓓ
25.	Ⓐ Ⓑ Ⓒ Ⓓ	50.	Ⓐ Ⓑ Ⓒ Ⓓ

V&S Publisher, Head Office: F-2/16 Ansari Road, Daryaganj, New Delhi-110002, Ph: 011-23240026-27, Email:info@vspublishers.com
Regional Office: 5-1-707/1, Brij Bhawan (Beside Central Bank of India Lane) Bank Street, Koti, Hyderabad-500 095, Ph: 040-24737290, Email: vspublishershyd@gmail.com
Branch: Jaywant Industrial Estate, 1st Floor–108, Tardeo Road Opposite Sobo Central Mall, Mumbai - 400 034, Ph: 022-23510736, Email: vspublishersmum@gmail.com

OMR ANSWER SHEET

1. NAME (IN ENGLISH CAPITAL LETTERS ONLY)

2. FATHER'S NAME (IN ENGLISH CAPITAL LETTERS ONLY)

Students must write and darken the respective circles completely for School Code, Class and Roll No. columns, othewise their Answer Sheets will not be evaluated.

3. SCHOOL CODE

Columns: [A–Z], [A–Z], [0–9], [0–9], [0–9], [0–9]

4. % of Marks | Grade

In Last Class

Percentage OR Grade

Percentage columns: [0–9], [0–9], [0–9]
Grade: [A–J]

5. CLASS

Columns: [0,1,2], [0,1,2,4,5,6,7,8,9,M,B]

6. ROLL NO.

Columns: [0–9], [0–9], [0–9]

7. GENDER

MALE ○
FEMALE ○

8. STREAM
(Only for Class XI and XII Students)

MATHEMATICS ○
BIOLOGY ○
OTHERS ○

9. MARK YOUR ANSWERS WITH HB PENCIL/BALL POINT PEN (BLUE/BLACK)

No.	A	B	C	D	No.	A	B	C	D
1.	Ⓐ	Ⓑ	Ⓒ	Ⓓ	26.	Ⓐ	Ⓑ	Ⓒ	Ⓓ
2.	Ⓐ	Ⓑ	Ⓒ	Ⓓ	27.	Ⓐ	Ⓑ	Ⓒ	Ⓓ
3.	Ⓐ	Ⓑ	Ⓒ	Ⓓ	28.	Ⓐ	Ⓑ	Ⓒ	Ⓓ
4.	Ⓐ	Ⓑ	Ⓒ	Ⓓ	29.	Ⓐ	Ⓑ	Ⓒ	Ⓓ
5.	Ⓐ	Ⓑ	Ⓒ	Ⓓ	30.	Ⓐ	Ⓑ	Ⓒ	Ⓓ
6.	Ⓐ	Ⓑ	Ⓒ	Ⓓ	31.	Ⓐ	Ⓑ	Ⓒ	Ⓓ
7.	Ⓐ	Ⓑ	Ⓒ	Ⓓ	32.	Ⓐ	Ⓑ	Ⓒ	Ⓓ
8.	Ⓐ	Ⓑ	Ⓒ	Ⓓ	33.	Ⓐ	Ⓑ	Ⓒ	Ⓓ
9.	Ⓐ	Ⓑ	Ⓒ	Ⓓ	34.	Ⓐ	Ⓑ	Ⓒ	Ⓓ
10.	Ⓐ	Ⓑ	Ⓒ	Ⓓ	35.	Ⓐ	Ⓑ	Ⓒ	Ⓓ
11.	Ⓐ	Ⓑ	Ⓒ	Ⓓ	36.	Ⓐ	Ⓑ	Ⓒ	Ⓓ
12.	Ⓐ	Ⓑ	Ⓒ	Ⓓ	37.	Ⓐ	Ⓑ	Ⓒ	Ⓓ
13.	Ⓐ	Ⓑ	Ⓒ	Ⓓ	38.	Ⓐ	Ⓑ	Ⓒ	Ⓓ
14.	Ⓐ	Ⓑ	Ⓒ	Ⓓ	39.	Ⓐ	Ⓑ	Ⓒ	Ⓓ
15.	Ⓐ	Ⓑ	Ⓒ	Ⓓ	40.	Ⓐ	Ⓑ	Ⓒ	Ⓓ
16.	Ⓐ	Ⓑ	Ⓒ	Ⓓ	41.	Ⓐ	Ⓑ	Ⓒ	Ⓓ
17.	Ⓐ	Ⓑ	Ⓒ	Ⓓ	42.	Ⓐ	Ⓑ	Ⓒ	Ⓓ
18.	Ⓐ	Ⓑ	Ⓒ	Ⓓ	43.	Ⓐ	Ⓑ	Ⓒ	Ⓓ
19.	Ⓐ	Ⓑ	Ⓒ	Ⓓ	44.	Ⓐ	Ⓑ	Ⓒ	Ⓓ
20.	Ⓐ	Ⓑ	Ⓒ	Ⓓ	45.	Ⓐ	Ⓑ	Ⓒ	Ⓓ
21.	Ⓐ	Ⓑ	Ⓒ	Ⓓ	46.	Ⓐ	Ⓑ	Ⓒ	Ⓓ
22.	Ⓐ	Ⓑ	Ⓒ	Ⓓ	47.	Ⓐ	Ⓑ	Ⓒ	Ⓓ
23.	Ⓐ	Ⓑ	Ⓒ	Ⓓ	48.	Ⓐ	Ⓑ	Ⓒ	Ⓓ
24.	Ⓐ	Ⓑ	Ⓒ	Ⓓ	49.	Ⓐ	Ⓑ	Ⓒ	Ⓓ
25.	Ⓐ	Ⓑ	Ⓒ	Ⓓ	50.	Ⓐ	Ⓑ	Ⓒ	Ⓓ

V&S Publisher, Head Office: F-2/16 Ansari Road, Daryaganj, New Delhi-110002, Ph: 011-23240026-27, Email:info@vspublishers.com
Regional Office: 5-1-707/1, Brij Bhawan (Beside Central Bank of India Lane) Bank Street, Koti, Hyderabad-500 095, Ph: 040-24737290, Email: vspublishershyd@gmail.com
Branch: Jaywant Industrial Estate, 1st Floor–108, Tardeo Road Opposite Sobo Central Mall, Mumbai - 400 034, Ph: 022-23510736, Email: vspublishersmum@gmail.com

OMR ANSWER SHEET

1. NAME (IN ENGLISH CAPITAL LETTERS ONLY)

2. FATHER'S NAME (IN ENGLISH CAPITAL LETTERS ONLY)

Students must write and darken the respective circles completely for School Code, Class and Roll No. columns, othewise their Answer Sheets will not be evaluated.

3. SCHOOL CODE

| | | 0 | 0 | 0 | 0 |
A A 0 0 0 0
B B 1 1 1 1
C C 2 2 2 2
D D 3 3 3 3
E E 4 4 4 4
F F 5 5 5 5
G G 6 6 6 6
H H 7 7 7 7
I I 8 8 8 8
J J 9 9 9 9
K K
L L

4. % of Marks | Grade
In Last Class

Percentage OR Grade

| | | |
0 0 0 A
1 1 1 B
2 2 2 C
3 3 3 D
4 4 4 E
5 5 5 F
6 6 6 G
7 7 7 H
8 8 8 I
9 9 9 J

M M
N N
O O
P P
Q Q
R R
S S
T T
U U
V V
W W
X X
Y Y
Z Z

5. CLASS

| | |
0 0
1 1
2 2
4
5
6
7
8
9
M
B

6. ROLL NO.

| | | |
0 0 0
1 1 1
2 2 2
3 3 3
4 4 4
5 5 5
6 6 6
7 7 7
8 8 8
9 9 9

7. GENDER

MALE ○
FEMALE ○

8. STREAM
(Only for Class XI and XII Students)

MATHEMATICS ○
BIOLOGY ○
OTHERS ○

9. MARK YOUR ANSWERS WITH HB PENCIL/BALL POINT PEN (BLUE/BLACK)

1.	Ⓐ Ⓑ Ⓒ Ⓓ	26.	Ⓐ Ⓑ Ⓒ Ⓓ
2.	Ⓐ Ⓑ Ⓒ Ⓓ	27.	Ⓐ Ⓑ Ⓒ Ⓓ
3.	Ⓐ Ⓑ Ⓒ Ⓓ	28.	Ⓐ Ⓑ Ⓒ Ⓓ
4.	Ⓐ Ⓑ Ⓒ Ⓓ	29.	Ⓐ Ⓑ Ⓒ Ⓓ
5.	Ⓐ Ⓑ Ⓒ Ⓓ	30.	Ⓐ Ⓑ Ⓒ Ⓓ
6.	Ⓐ Ⓑ Ⓒ Ⓓ	31.	Ⓐ Ⓑ Ⓒ Ⓓ
7.	Ⓐ Ⓑ Ⓒ Ⓓ	32.	Ⓐ Ⓑ Ⓒ Ⓓ
8.	Ⓐ Ⓑ Ⓒ Ⓓ	33.	Ⓐ Ⓑ Ⓒ Ⓓ
9.	Ⓐ Ⓑ Ⓒ Ⓓ	34.	Ⓐ Ⓑ Ⓒ Ⓓ
10.	Ⓐ Ⓑ Ⓒ Ⓓ	35.	Ⓐ Ⓑ Ⓒ Ⓓ
11.	Ⓐ Ⓑ Ⓒ Ⓓ	36.	Ⓐ Ⓑ Ⓒ Ⓓ
12.	Ⓐ Ⓑ Ⓒ Ⓓ	37.	Ⓐ Ⓑ Ⓒ Ⓓ
13.	Ⓐ Ⓑ Ⓒ Ⓓ	38.	Ⓐ Ⓑ Ⓒ Ⓓ
14.	Ⓐ Ⓑ Ⓒ Ⓓ	39.	Ⓐ Ⓑ Ⓒ Ⓓ
15.	Ⓐ Ⓑ Ⓒ Ⓓ	40.	Ⓐ Ⓑ Ⓒ Ⓓ
16.	Ⓐ Ⓑ Ⓒ Ⓓ	41.	Ⓐ Ⓑ Ⓒ Ⓓ
17.	Ⓐ Ⓑ Ⓒ Ⓓ	42.	Ⓐ Ⓑ Ⓒ Ⓓ
18.	Ⓐ Ⓑ Ⓒ Ⓓ	43.	Ⓐ Ⓑ Ⓒ Ⓓ
19.	Ⓐ Ⓑ Ⓒ Ⓓ	44.	Ⓐ Ⓑ Ⓒ Ⓓ
20.	Ⓐ Ⓑ Ⓒ Ⓓ	45.	Ⓐ Ⓑ Ⓒ Ⓓ
21.	Ⓐ Ⓑ Ⓒ Ⓓ	46.	Ⓐ Ⓑ Ⓒ Ⓓ
22.	Ⓐ Ⓑ Ⓒ Ⓓ	47.	Ⓐ Ⓑ Ⓒ Ⓓ
23.	Ⓐ Ⓑ Ⓒ Ⓓ	48.	Ⓐ Ⓑ Ⓒ Ⓓ
24.	Ⓐ Ⓑ Ⓒ Ⓓ	49.	Ⓐ Ⓑ Ⓒ Ⓓ
25.	Ⓐ Ⓑ Ⓒ Ⓓ	50.	Ⓐ Ⓑ Ⓒ Ⓓ

V&S Publisher, Head Office: F-2/16 Ansari Road, Daryaganj, New Delhi-110002, Ph: 011-23240026-27, Email:info@vspublishers.com
Regional Office: 5-1-707/1, Brij Bhawan (Beside Central Bank of India Lane) Bank Street, Koti, Hyderabad-500 095, Ph: 040-24737290, Email: vspublishershyd@gmail.com
Branch: Jaywant Industrial Estate, 1st Floor–108, Tardeo Road Opposite Sobo Central Mall, Mumbai - 400 034, Ph: 022-23510736, Email: vspublishersmum@gmail.com

OMR ANSWER SHEET

1. NAME (IN ENGLISH CAPITAL LETTERS ONLY)

2. FATHER'S NAME (IN ENGLISH CAPITAL LETTERS ONLY)

Students must write and darken the respective circles completely for School Code, Class and Roll No. columns, othewise their Answer Sheets will not be evaluated.

3. SCHOOL CODE

4. % of Marks | Grade
In Last Class

Percentage OR Grade

5. CLASS

6. ROLL NO.

7. GENDER

MALE ◯

FEMALE ◯

8. STREAM
(Only for Class XI and XII Students)

MATHEMATICS ◯
BIOLOGY ◯
OTHERS

9. MARK YOUR ANSWERS WITH HB PENCIL/BALL POINT PEN (BLUE/BLACK)

No.	A B C D	No.	A B C D
1.	Ⓐ Ⓑ Ⓒ Ⓓ	26.	Ⓐ Ⓑ Ⓒ Ⓓ
2.	Ⓐ Ⓑ Ⓒ Ⓓ	27.	Ⓐ Ⓑ Ⓒ Ⓓ
3.	Ⓐ Ⓑ Ⓒ Ⓓ	28.	Ⓐ Ⓑ Ⓒ Ⓓ
4.	Ⓐ Ⓑ Ⓒ Ⓓ	29.	Ⓐ Ⓑ Ⓒ Ⓓ
5.	Ⓐ Ⓑ Ⓒ Ⓓ	30.	Ⓐ Ⓑ Ⓒ Ⓓ
6.	Ⓐ Ⓑ Ⓒ Ⓓ	31.	Ⓐ Ⓑ Ⓒ Ⓓ
7.	Ⓐ Ⓑ Ⓒ Ⓓ	32.	Ⓐ Ⓑ Ⓒ Ⓓ
8.	Ⓐ Ⓑ Ⓒ Ⓓ	33.	Ⓐ Ⓑ Ⓒ Ⓓ
9.	Ⓐ Ⓑ Ⓒ Ⓓ	34.	Ⓐ Ⓑ Ⓒ Ⓓ
10.	Ⓐ Ⓑ Ⓒ Ⓓ	35.	Ⓐ Ⓑ Ⓒ Ⓓ
11.	Ⓐ Ⓑ Ⓒ Ⓓ	36.	Ⓐ Ⓑ Ⓒ Ⓓ
12.	Ⓐ Ⓑ Ⓒ Ⓓ	37.	Ⓐ Ⓑ Ⓒ Ⓓ
13.	Ⓐ Ⓑ Ⓒ Ⓓ	38.	Ⓐ Ⓑ Ⓒ Ⓓ
14.	Ⓐ Ⓑ Ⓒ Ⓓ	39.	Ⓐ Ⓑ Ⓒ Ⓓ
15.	Ⓐ Ⓑ Ⓒ Ⓓ	40.	Ⓐ Ⓑ Ⓒ Ⓓ
16.	Ⓐ Ⓑ Ⓒ Ⓓ	41.	Ⓐ Ⓑ Ⓒ Ⓓ
17.	Ⓐ Ⓑ Ⓒ Ⓓ	42.	Ⓐ Ⓑ Ⓒ Ⓓ
18.	Ⓐ Ⓑ Ⓒ Ⓓ	43.	Ⓐ Ⓑ Ⓒ Ⓓ
19.	Ⓐ Ⓑ Ⓒ Ⓓ	44.	Ⓐ Ⓑ Ⓒ Ⓓ
20.	Ⓐ Ⓑ Ⓒ Ⓓ	45.	Ⓐ Ⓑ Ⓒ Ⓓ
21.	Ⓐ Ⓑ Ⓒ Ⓓ	46.	Ⓐ Ⓑ Ⓒ Ⓓ
22.	Ⓐ Ⓑ Ⓒ Ⓓ	47.	Ⓐ Ⓑ Ⓒ Ⓓ
23.	Ⓐ Ⓑ Ⓒ Ⓓ	48.	Ⓐ Ⓑ Ⓒ Ⓓ
24.	Ⓐ Ⓑ Ⓒ Ⓓ	49.	Ⓐ Ⓑ Ⓒ Ⓓ
25.	Ⓐ Ⓑ Ⓒ Ⓓ	50.	Ⓐ Ⓑ Ⓒ Ⓓ

V&S Publisher, Head Office: F-2/16 Ansari Road, Daryaganj, New Delhi-110002, Ph: 011-23240026-27, Email:info@vspublishers.com
Regional Office: 5-1-707/1, Brij Bhawan (Beside Central Bank of India Lane) Bank Street, Koti, Hyderabad-500 095, Ph: 040-24737290, Email: vspublishershyd@gmail.com
Branch: Jaywant Industrial Estate, 1st Floor–108, Tardeo Road Opposite Sobo Central Mall, Mumbai - 400 034, Ph: 022-23510736, Email: vspublishersmum@gmail.com

OMR ANSWER SHEET

1. NAME (IN ENGLISH CAPITAL LETTERS ONLY)

2. FATHER'S NAME (IN ENGLISH CAPITAL LETTERS ONLY)

Students must write and darken the respective circles completely for School Code, Class and Roll No. columns, othewise their Answer Sheets will not be evaluated.

3. SCHOOL CODE

(A) (A) (0) (0) (0) (0)
(B) (B) (1) (1) (1) (1)
(C) (C) (2) (2) (2) (2)
(D) (D) (3) (3) (3) (3)
(E) (E) (4) (4) (4) (4)
(F) (F) (5) (5) (5) (5)
(G) (G) (6) (6) (6) (6)
(H) (H) (7) (7) (7) (7)
(I) (I) (8) (8) (8) (8)
(J) (J) (9) (9) (9) (9)
(K) (K)
(L) (L)
(M) (M)
(N) (N)
(O) (O)
(P) (P)
(Q) (Q)
(R) (R)
(S) (S)
(T) (T)
(U) (U)
(V) (V)
(W) (W)
(X) (X)
(Y) (Y)
(Z) (Z)

4. % of Marks / Grade

In Last Class

Percentage	OR	Grade

(0) (0) (0) — (A)
(1) (1) (1) — (B)
(2) (2) (2) — (C)
(3) (3) (3) — (D)
(4) (4) (4) — (E)
(5) (5) (5) — (F)
(6) (6) (6) — (G)
(7) (7) (7) — (H)
(8) (8) (8) — (I)
(9) (9) (9) — (J)

5. CLASS

(0) (0)
(1) (1)
(2) (2)
    (4)
    (5)
    (6)
    (7)
    (8)
    (9)
    (M)
    (B)

6. ROLL NO.

(0) (0) (0)
(1) (1) (1)
(2) (2) (2)
(3) (3) (3)
(4) (4) (4)
(5) (5) (5)
(6) (6) (6)
(7) (7) (7)
(8) (8) (8)
(9) (9) (9)

7. GENDER

MALE ○
FEMALE ○

8. STREAM
(Only for Class XI and XII Students)

MATHEMATICS ○
BIOLOGY ○
OTHERS ○

9. MARK YOUR ANSWERS WITH HB PENCIL/BALL POINT PEN (BLUE/BLACK)

No.					No.				
1.	(A)	(B)	(C)	(D)	26.	(A)	(B)	(C)	(D)
2.	(A)	(B)	(C)	(D)	27.	(A)	(B)	(C)	(D)
3.	(A)	(B)	(C)	(D)	28.	(A)	(B)	(C)	(D)
4.	(A)	(B)	(C)	(D)	29.	(A)	(B)	(C)	(D)
5.	(A)	(B)	(C)	(D)	30.	(A)	(B)	(C)	(D)
6.	(A)	(B)	(C)	(D)	31.	(A)	(B)	(C)	(D)
7.	(A)	(B)	(C)	(D)	32.	(A)	(B)	(C)	(D)
8.	(A)	(B)	(C)	(D)	33.	(A)	(B)	(C)	(D)
9.	(A)	(B)	(C)	(D)	34.	(A)	(B)	(C)	(D)
10.	(A)	(B)	(C)	(D)	35.	(A)	(B)	(C)	(D)
11.	(A)	(B)	(C)	(D)	36.	(A)	(B)	(C)	(D)
12.	(A)	(B)	(C)	(D)	37.	(A)	(B)	(C)	(D)
13.	(A)	(B)	(C)	(D)	38.	(A)	(B)	(C)	(D)
14.	(A)	(B)	(C)	(D)	39.	(A)	(B)	(C)	(D)
15.	(A)	(B)	(C)	(D)	40.	(A)	(B)	(C)	(D)
16.	(A)	(B)	(C)	(D)	41.	(A)	(B)	(C)	(D)
17.	(A)	(B)	(C)	(D)	42.	(A)	(B)	(C)	(D)
18.	(A)	(B)	(C)	(D)	43.	(A)	(B)	(C)	(D)
19.	(A)	(B)	(C)	(D)	44.	(A)	(B)	(C)	(D)
20.	(A)	(B)	(C)	(D)	45.	(A)	(B)	(C)	(D)
21.	(A)	(B)	(C)	(D)	46.	(A)	(B)	(C)	(D)
22.	(A)	(B)	(C)	(D)	47.	(A)	(B)	(C)	(D)
23.	(A)	(B)	(C)	(D)	48.	(A)	(B)	(C)	(D)
24.	(A)	(B)	(C)	(D)	49.	(A)	(B)	(C)	(D)
25.	(A)	(B)	(C)	(D)	50.	(A)	(B)	(C)	(D)

V&S Publisher, Head Office: F-2/16 Ansari Road, Daryaganj, New Delhi-110002, Ph: 011-23240026-27, Email:info@vspublishers.com
Regional Office: 5-1-707/1, Brij Bhawan (Beside Central Bank of India Lane) Bank Street, Koti, Hyderabad-500 095, Ph: 040-24737290, Email: vspublishershyd@gmail.com
Branch: Jaywant Industrial Estate, 1st Floor–108, Tardeo Road Opposite Sobo Central Mall, Mumbai - 400 034, Ph: 022-23510736, Email: vspublishersmum@gmail.com

OMR ANSWER SHEET

1. NAME (IN ENGLISH CAPITAL LETTERS ONLY)

2. FATHER'S NAME (IN ENGLISH CAPITAL LETTERS ONLY)

Students must write and darken the respective circles completely for School Code, Class and Roll No. columns, othewise their Answer Sheets will not be evaluated.

3. SCHOOL CODE

(A) (A) (0) (0) (0) (0)
(B) (B) (1) (1) (1) (1)
(C) (C) (2) (2) (2) (2)
(D) (D) (3) (3) (3) (3)
(E) (E) (4) (4) (4) (4)
(F) (F) (5) (5) (5) (5)
(G) (G) (6) (6) (6) (6)
(H) (H) (7) (7) (7) (7)
(I) (I) (8) (8) (8) (8)
(J) (J) (9) (9) (9) (9)
(K) (K)
(L) (L)
(M) (M)
(N) (N)
(O) (O)
(P) (P)
(Q) (Q)
(R) (R)
(S) (S)
(T) (T)
(U) (U)
(V) (V)
(W) (W)
(X) (X)
(Y) (Y)
(Z) (Z)

4. % of Marks | Grade

In Last Class

Percentage	OR	Grade

(0) (0) (0) — (A)
(1) (1) (1) — (B)
(2) (2) (2) — (C)
(3) (3) (3) — (D)
(4) (4) (4) — (E)
(5) (5) (5) — (F)
(6) (6) (6) — (G)
(7) (7) (7) — (H)
(8) (8) (8) — (I)
(9) (9) (9) — (J)

5. CLASS

(0) (0)
(1) (1)
(2) (2)
(4)
(5)
(6)
(7)
(8)
(9)
(M)
(B)

6. ROLL NO.

(0) (0) (0)
(1) (1) (1)
(2) (2) (2)
(3) (3) (3)
(4) (4) (4)
(5) (5) (5)
(6) (6) (6)
(7) (7) (7)
(8) (8) (8)
(9) (9) (9)

7. GENDER

MALE ○
FEMALE ○

8. STREAM
(Only for Class XI and XII Students)

MATHEMATICS ○
BIOLOGY ○
OTHERS ○

9. MARK YOUR ANSWERS WITH HB PENCIL/BALL POINT PEN (BLUE/BLACK)

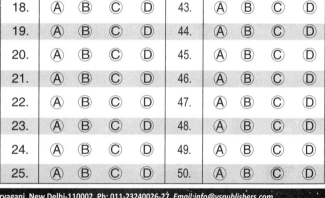

1. (A) (B) (C) (D)	26. (A) (B) (C) (D)
2. (A) (B) (C) (D)	27. (A) (B) (C) (D)
3. (A) (B) (C) (D)	28. (A) (B) (C) (D)
4. (A) (B) (C) (D)	29. (A) (B) (C) (D)
5. (A) (B) (C) (D)	30. (A) (B) (C) (D)
6. (A) (B) (C) (D)	31. (A) (B) (C) (D)
7. (A) (B) (C) (D)	32. (A) (B) (C) (D)
8. (A) (B) (C) (D)	33. (A) (B) (C) (D)
9. (A) (B) (C) (D)	34. (A) (B) (C) (D)
10. (A) (B) (C) (D)	35. (A) (B) (C) (D)
11. (A) (B) (C) (D)	36. (A) (B) (C) (D)
12. (A) (B) (C) (D)	37. (A) (B) (C) (D)
13. (A) (B) (C) (D)	38. (A) (B) (C) (D)
14. (A) (B) (C) (D)	39. (A) (B) (C) (D)
15. (A) (B) (C) (D)	40. (A) (B) (C) (D)
16. (A) (B) (C) (D)	41. (A) (B) (C) (D)
17. (A) (B) (C) (D)	42. (A) (B) (C) (D)
18. (A) (B) (C) (D)	43. (A) (B) (C) (D)
19. (A) (B) (C) (D)	44. (A) (B) (C) (D)
20. (A) (B) (C) (D)	45. (A) (B) (C) (D)
21. (A) (B) (C) (D)	46. (A) (B) (C) (D)
22. (A) (B) (C) (D)	47. (A) (B) (C) (D)
23. (A) (B) (C) (D)	48. (A) (B) (C) (D)
24. (A) (B) (C) (D)	49. (A) (B) (C) (D)
25. (A) (B) (C) (D)	50. (A) (B) (C) (D)

V&S Publisher, Head Office: F-2/16 Ansari Road, Daryaganj, New Delhi-110002, Ph: 011-23240026-27, Email:info@vspublishers.com
Regional Office: 5-1-707/1, Brij Bhawan (Beside Central Bank of India Lane) Bank Street, Koti, Hyderabad-500 095, Ph: 040-24737290, Email: vspublishershyd@gmail.com
Branch: Jaywant Industrial Estate, 1st Floor–108, Tardeo Road Opposite Sobo Central Mall, Mumbai - 400 034, Ph: 022-23510736, Email: vspublishersmum@gmail.com

OMR ANSWER SHEET

1. NAME (IN ENGLISH CAPITAL LETTERS ONLY)

2. FATHER'S NAME (IN ENGLISH CAPITAL LETTERS ONLY)

Students must write and darken the respective circles completely for School Code, Class and Roll No. columns, othewise their Answer Sheets will not be evaluated.

3. SCHOOL CODE

(A)(B)(C)(D)(E)(F)(G)(H)(I)(J)(K)(L)(M)(N)(O)(P)(Q)(R)(S)(T)(U)(V)(W)(X)(Y)(Z)

(A)(B)(C)(D)(E)(F)(G)(H)(I)(J)(K)(L)(M)(N)(O)(P)(Q)(R)(S)(T)(U)(V)(W)(X)(Y)(Z)

(0)(1)(2)(3)(4)(5)(6)(7)(8)(9)

(0)(1)(2)(3)(4)(5)(6)(7)(8)(9)

(0)(1)(2)(3)(4)(5)(6)(7)(8)(9)

(0)(1)(2)(3)(4)(5)(6)(7)(8)(9)

4. % of Marks | Grade
In Last Class

Percentage	OR	Grade

(0)(0)(0) (1)(1)(1) (2)(2)(2) (3)(3)(3) (4)(4)(4) (5)(5)(5) (6)(6)(6) (7)(7)(7) (8)(8)(8) (9)(9)(9)

(A)(B)(C)(D)(E)(F)(G)(H)(I)(J)

5. CLASS

(0)(1)(2)(4)(5)(6)(7)(8)(9)(M)(B)

(0)(1)(2)

6. ROLL NO.

(0)(1)(2)(3)(4)(5)(6)(7)(8)(9)

(0)(1)(2)(3)(4)(5)(6)(7)(8)(9)

(0)(1)(2)(3)(4)(5)(6)(7)(8)(9)

7. GENDER

MALE ◯
FEMALE ◯

8. STREAM
(Only for Class XI and XII Students)

MATHEMATICS ◯
BIOLOGY ◯
OTHERS ◯

9. MARK YOUR ANSWERS WITH HB PENCIL/BALL POINT PEN (BLUE/BLACK)

1. (A) (B) (C) (D) 26. (A) (B) (C) (D)
2. (A) (B) (C) (D) 27. (A) (B) (C) (D)
3. (A) (B) (C) (D) 28. (A) (B) (C) (D)
4. (A) (B) (C) (D) 29. (A) (B) (C) (D)
5. (A) (B) (C) (D) 30. (A) (B) (C) (D)
6. (A) (B) (C) (D) 31. (A) (B) (C) (D)
7. (A) (B) (C) (D) 32. (A) (B) (C) (D)
8. (A) (B) (C) (D) 33. (A) (B) (C) (D)
9. (A) (B) (C) (D) 34. (A) (B) (C) (D)
10. (A) (B) (C) (D) 35. (A) (B) (C) (D)
11. (A) (B) (C) (D) 36. (A) (B) (C) (D)
12. (A) (B) (C) (D) 37. (A) (B) (C) (D)
13. (A) (B) (C) (D) 38. (A) (B) (C) (D)
14. (A) (B) (C) (D) 39. (A) (B) (C) (D)
15. (A) (B) (C) (D) 40. (A) (B) (C) (D)
16. (A) (B) (C) (D) 41. (A) (B) (C) (D)
17. (A) (B) (C) (D) 42. (A) (B) (C) (D)
18. (A) (B) (C) (D) 43. (A) (B) (C) (D)
19. (A) (B) (C) (D) 44. (A) (B) (C) (D)
20. (A) (B) (C) (D) 45. (A) (B) (C) (D)
21. (A) (B) (C) (D) 46. (A) (B) (C) (D)
22. (A) (B) (C) (D) 47. (A) (B) (C) (D)
23. (A) (B) (C) (D) 48. (A) (B) (C) (D)
24. (A) (B) (C) (D) 49. (A) (B) (C) (D)
25. (A) (B) (C) (D) 50. (A) (B) (C) (D)

V&S Publisher, Head Office: F-2/16 Ansari Road, Daryaganj, New Delhi-110002, Ph: 011-23240026-27, Email:info@vspublishers.com
Regional Office: 5-1-707/1, Brij Bhawan (Beside Central Bank of India Lane) Bank Street, Koti, Hyderabad-500 095, Ph: 040-24737290, Email: vspublishershyd@gmail.com
Branch: Jaywant Industrial Estate, 1st Floor–108, Tardeo Road Opposite Sobo Central Mall, Mumbai - 400 034, Ph: 022-23510736, Email: vspublishersmum@gmail.com

OMR ANSWER SHEET

1. NAME (IN ENGLISH CAPITAL LETTERS ONLY)

2. FATHER'S NAME (IN ENGLISH CAPITAL LETTERS ONLY)

Students must write and darken the respective circles completely for School Code, Class and Roll No. columns, otherwise their Answer Sheets will not be evaluated.

3. SCHOOL CODE

(A) (A) (0) (0) (0) (0)
(B) (B) (1) (1) (1) (1)
(C) (C) (2) (2) (2) (2)
(D) (D) (3) (3) (3) (3)
(E) (E) (4) (4) (4) (4)
(F) (F) (5) (5) (5) (5)
(G) (G) (6) (6) (6) (6)
(H) (H) (7) (7) (7) (7)
(I) (I) (8) (8) (8) (8)
(J) (J) (9) (9) (9) (9)
(K) (K)
(L) (L)
(M) (M)
(N) (N)
(O) (O)
(P) (P)
(Q) (Q)
(R) (R)
(S) (S)
(T) (T)
(U) (U)
(V) (V)
(W) (W)
(X) (X)
(Y) (Y)
(Z) (Z)

4. % of Marks | Grade

In Last Class

Percentage OR Grade

(0) (0) (0) — (A)
(1) (1) (1) — (B)
(2) (2) (2) — (C)
(3) (3) (3) — (D)
(4) (4) (4) — (E)
(5) (5) (5) — (F)
(6) (6) (6) — (G)
(7) (7) (7) — (H)
(8) (8) (8) — (I)
(9) (9) (9) — (J)

5. CLASS

(0) (0)
(1) (1)
(2) (2)
     (4)
     (5)
     (6)
     (7)
     (8)
     (9)
     (M)
     (B)

6. ROLL NO.

(0) (0) (0)
(1) (1) (1)
(2) (2) (2)
(3) (3) (3)
(4) (4) (4)
(5) (5) (5)
(6) (6) (6)
(7) (7) (7)
(8) (8) (8)
(9) (9) (9)

7. GENDER

MALE ○
FEMALE ○

8. STREAM
(Only for Class XI and XII Students)

MATHEMATICS ○
BIOLOGY ○
OTHERS ○

9. MARK YOUR ANSWERS WITH HB PENCIL/BALL POINT PEN (BLUE/BLACK)

No.	A B C D	No.	A B C D
1.	(A) (B) (C) (D)	26.	(A) (B) (C) (D)
2.	(A) (B) (C) (D)	27.	(A) (B) (C) (D)
3.	(A) (B) (C) (D)	28.	(A) (B) (C) (D)
4.	(A) (B) (C) (D)	29.	(A) (B) (C) (D)
5.	(A) (B) (C) (D)	30.	(A) (B) (C) (D)
6.	(A) (B) (C) (D)	31.	(A) (B) (C) (D)
7.	(A) (B) (C) (D)	32.	(A) (B) (C) (D)
8.	(A) (B) (C) (D)	33.	(A) (B) (C) (D)
9.	(A) (B) (C) (D)	34.	(A) (B) (C) (D)
10.	(A) (B) (C) (D)	35.	(A) (B) (C) (D)
11.	(A) (B) (C) (D)	36.	(A) (B) (C) (D)
12.	(A) (B) (C) (D)	37.	(A) (B) (C) (D)
13.	(A) (B) (C) (D)	38.	(A) (B) (C) (D)
14.	(A) (B) (C) (D)	39.	(A) (B) (C) (D)
15.	(A) (B) (C) (D)	40.	(A) (B) (C) (D)
16.	(A) (B) (C) (D)	41.	(A) (B) (C) (D)
17.	(A) (B) (C) (D)	42.	(A) (B) (C) (D)
18.	(A) (B) (C) (D)	43.	(A) (B) (C) (D)
19.	(A) (B) (C) (D)	44.	(A) (B) (C) (D)
20.	(A) (B) (C) (D)	45.	(A) (B) (C) (D)
21.	(A) (B) (C) (D)	46.	(A) (B) (C) (D)
22.	(A) (B) (C) (D)	47.	(A) (B) (C) (D)
23.	(A) (B) (C) (D)	48.	(A) (B) (C) (D)
24.	(A) (B) (C) (D)	49.	(A) (B) (C) (D)
25.	(A) (B) (C) (D)	50.	(A) (B) (C) (D)

V&S Publisher, Head Office: F-2/16 Ansari Road, Daryaganj, New Delhi-110002, Ph: 011-23240026-27, Email:info@vspublishers.com
Regional Office: 5-1-707/1, Brij Bhawan (Beside Central Bank of India Lane) Bank Street, Koti, Hyderabad-500 095, Ph: 040-24737290, Email: vspublishershyd@gmail.com
Branch: Jaywant Industrial Estate, 1st Floor–108, Tardeo Road Opposite Sobo Central Mall, Mumbai - 400 034, Ph: 022-23510736, Email: vspublishersmum@gmail.com

OMR ANSWER SHEET

1. NAME (IN ENGLISH CAPITAL LETTERS ONLY)

2. FATHER'S NAME (IN ENGLISH CAPITAL LETTERS ONLY)

Students must write and darken the respective circles completely for School Code, Class and Roll No. columns, othewise their Answer Sheets will not be evaluated.

3. SCHOOL CODE

(A)(B)(C)(D)(E)(F)(G)(H)(I)(J)(K)(L)(M)(N)(O)(P)(Q)(R)(S)(T)(U)(V)(W)(X)(Y)(Z)

(0)(1)(2)(3)(4)(5)(6)(7)(8)(9)

4. % of Marks | Grade

In Last Class

Percentage	OR	Grade

(0)(1)(2)(3)(4)(5)(6)(7)(8)(9)

(A)(B)(C)(D)(E)(F)(G)(H)(I)(J)

5. CLASS

(0)(1)(2)(4)(5)(6)(7)(8)(9)(M)(B)

6. ROLL NO.

(0)(1)(2)(3)(4)(5)(6)(7)(8)(9)

7. GENDER

MALE ○
FEMALE ○

8. STREAM
(Only for Class XI and XII Students)

MATHEMATICS ○
BIOLOGY ○
OTHERS ○

9. MARK YOUR ANSWERS WITH HB PENCIL/BALL POINT PEN (BLUE/BLACK)

1. (A) (B) (C) (D)   26. (A) (B) (C) (D)
2. (A) (B) (C) (D)   27. (A) (B) (C) (D)
3. (A) (B) (C) (D)   28. (A) (B) (C) (D)
4. (A) (B) (C) (D)   29. (A) (B) (C) (D)
5. (A) (B) (C) (D)   30. (A) (B) (C) (D)
6. (A) (B) (C) (D)   31. (A) (B) (C) (D)
7. (A) (B) (C) (D)   32. (A) (B) (C) (D)
8. (A) (B) (C) (D)   33. (A) (B) (C) (D)
9. (A) (B) (C) (D)   34. (A) (B) (C) (D)
10. (A) (B) (C) (D)   35. (A) (B) (C) (D)
11. (A) (B) (C) (D)   36. (A) (B) (C) (D)
12. (A) (B) (C) (D)   37. (A) (B) (C) (D)
13. (A) (B) (C) (D)   38. (A) (B) (C) (D)
14. (A) (B) (C) (D)   39. (A) (B) (C) (D)
15. (A) (B) (C) (D)   40. (A) (B) (C) (D)
16. (A) (B) (C) (D)   41. (A) (B) (C) (D)
17. (A) (B) (C) (D)   42. (A) (B) (C) (D)
18. (A) (B) (C) (D)   43. (A) (B) (C) (D)
19. (A) (B) (C) (D)   44. (A) (B) (C) (D)
20. (A) (B) (C) (D)   45. (A) (B) (C) (D)
21. (A) (B) (C) (D)   46. (A) (B) (C) (D)
22. (A) (B) (C) (D)   47. (A) (B) (C) (D)
23. (A) (B) (C) (D)   48. (A) (B) (C) (D)
24. (A) (B) (C) (D)   49. (A) (B) (C) (D)
25. (A) (B) (C) (D)   50. (A) (B) (C) (D)

V&S Publisher, Head Office: F-2/16 Ansari Road, Daryaganj, New Delhi-110002, Ph: 011-23240026-27, Email:info@vspublishers.com
Regional Office: 5-1-707/1, Brij Bhawan (Beside Central Bank of India Lane) Bank Street, Koti, Hyderabad-500 095, Ph: 040-24737290, Email: vspublishershyd@gmail.com
Branch: Jaywant Industrial Estate, 1st Floor–108, Tardeo Road Opposite Sobo Central Mall, Mumbai - 400 034, Ph: 022-23510736, Email: vspublishersmum@gmail.com

OMR ANSWER SHEET

1. NAME (IN ENGLISH CAPITAL LETTERS ONLY)

2. FATHER'S NAME (IN ENGLISH CAPITAL LETTERS ONLY)

Students must write and darken the respective circles completely for School Code, Class and Roll No. columns, othewise their Answer Sheets will not be evaluated.

3. SCHOOL CODE

A–Z	A–Z	0–9	0–9	0–9	0–9

4. % of Marks / Grade

In Last Class

Percentage OR Grade

Percentage			Grade
0–9	0–9	0–9	A–J

5. CLASS

0, 1, 2	0, 1, 2, 4, 5, 6, 7, 8, 9, M, B

6. ROLL NO.

0–9	0–9	0–9

7. GENDER

MALE ○

FEMALE ○

8. STREAM
(Only for Class XI and XII Students)

MATHEMATICS ○

BIOLOGY ○

OTHERS ○

9. MARK YOUR ANSWERS WITH HB PENCIL/BALL POINT PEN (BLUE/BLACK)

No.					No.				
1.	A	B	C	D	26.	A	B	C	D
2.	A	B	C	D	27.	A	B	C	D
3.	A	B	C	D	28.	A	B	C	D
4.	A	B	C	D	29.	A	B	C	D
5.	A	B	C	D	30.	A	B	C	D
6.	A	B	C	D	31.	A	B	C	D
7.	A	B	C	D	32.	A	B	C	D
8.	A	B	C	D	33.	A	B	C	D
9.	A	B	C	D	34.	A	B	C	D
10.	A	B	C	D	35.	A	B	C	D
11.	A	B	C	D	36.	A	B	C	D
12.	A	B	C	D	37.	A	B	C	D
13.	A	B	C	D	38.	A	B	C	D
14.	A	B	C	D	39.	A	B	C	D
15.	A	B	C	D	40.	A	B	C	D
16.	A	B	C	D	41.	A	B	C	D
17.	A	B	C	D	42.	A	B	C	D
18.	A	B	C	D	43.	A	B	C	D
19.	A	B	C	D	44.	A	B	C	D
20.	A	B	C	D	45.	A	B	C	D
21.	A	B	C	D	46.	A	B	C	D
22.	A	B	C	D	47.	A	B	C	D
23.	A	B	C	D	48.	A	B	C	D
24.	A	B	C	D	49.	A	B	C	D
25.	A	B	C	D	50.	A	B	C	D

V&S Publisher, Head Office: F-2/16 Ansari Road, Daryaganj, New Delhi-110002, Ph: 011-23240026-27, Email:info@vspublishers.com
Regional Office: 5-1-707/1, Brij Bhawan (Beside Central Bank of India Lane) Bank Street, Koti, Hyderabad-500 095, Ph: 040-24737290, Email: vspublishershyd@gmail.com
Branch: Jaywant Industrial Estate, 1st Floor–108, Tardeo Road Opposite Sobo Central Mall, Mumbai - 400 034, Ph: 022-23510736, Email: vspublishersmum@gmail.com

OMR ANSWER SHEET

1. NAME (IN ENGLISH CAPITAL LETTERS ONLY)

2. FATHER'S NAME (IN ENGLISH CAPITAL LETTERS ONLY)

Students must write and darken the respective circles completely for School Code, Class and Roll No. columns, othewise their Answer Sheets will not be evaluated.

3. SCHOOL CODE

4. % of Marks | Grade

In Last Class

Percentage OR Grade

5. CLASS

6. ROLL NO.

7. GENDER

MALE ⚪

FEMALE ⚪

8. STREAM
(Only for Class XI and XII Students)

MATHEMATICS ⚪
BIOLOGY ⚪
OTHERS ⚪

9. MARK YOUR ANSWERS WITH HB PENCIL/BALL POINT PEN (BLUE/BLACK)

1.	Ⓐ	Ⓑ	Ⓒ	Ⓓ	26.	Ⓐ	Ⓑ	Ⓒ	Ⓓ
2.	Ⓐ	Ⓑ	Ⓒ	Ⓓ	27.	Ⓐ	Ⓑ	Ⓒ	Ⓓ
3.	Ⓐ	Ⓑ	Ⓒ	Ⓓ	28.	Ⓐ	Ⓑ	Ⓒ	Ⓓ
4.	Ⓐ	Ⓑ	Ⓒ	Ⓓ	29.	Ⓐ	Ⓑ	Ⓒ	Ⓓ
5.	Ⓐ	Ⓑ	Ⓒ	Ⓓ	30.	Ⓐ	Ⓑ	Ⓒ	Ⓓ
6.	Ⓐ	Ⓑ	Ⓒ	Ⓓ	31.	Ⓐ	Ⓑ	Ⓒ	Ⓓ
7.	Ⓐ	Ⓑ	Ⓒ	Ⓓ	32.	Ⓐ	Ⓑ	Ⓒ	Ⓓ
8.	Ⓐ	Ⓑ	Ⓒ	Ⓓ	33.	Ⓐ	Ⓑ	Ⓒ	Ⓓ
9.	Ⓐ	Ⓑ	Ⓒ	Ⓓ	34.	Ⓐ	Ⓑ	Ⓒ	Ⓓ
10.	Ⓐ	Ⓑ	Ⓒ	Ⓓ	35.	Ⓐ	Ⓑ	Ⓒ	Ⓓ
11.	Ⓐ	Ⓑ	Ⓒ	Ⓓ	36.	Ⓐ	Ⓑ	Ⓒ	Ⓓ
12.	Ⓐ	Ⓑ	Ⓒ	Ⓓ	37.	Ⓐ	Ⓑ	Ⓒ	Ⓓ
13.	Ⓐ	Ⓑ	Ⓒ	Ⓓ	38.	Ⓐ	Ⓑ	Ⓒ	Ⓓ
14.	Ⓐ	Ⓑ	Ⓒ	Ⓓ	39.	Ⓐ	Ⓑ	Ⓒ	Ⓓ
15.	Ⓐ	Ⓑ	Ⓒ	Ⓓ	40.	Ⓐ	Ⓑ	Ⓒ	Ⓓ
16.	Ⓐ	Ⓑ	Ⓒ	Ⓓ	41.	Ⓐ	Ⓑ	Ⓒ	Ⓓ
17.	Ⓐ	Ⓑ	Ⓒ	Ⓓ	42.	Ⓐ	Ⓑ	Ⓒ	Ⓓ
18.	Ⓐ	Ⓑ	Ⓒ	Ⓓ	43.	Ⓐ	Ⓑ	Ⓒ	Ⓓ
19.	Ⓐ	Ⓑ	Ⓒ	Ⓓ	44.	Ⓐ	Ⓑ	Ⓒ	Ⓓ
20.	Ⓐ	Ⓑ	Ⓒ	Ⓓ	45.	Ⓐ	Ⓑ	Ⓒ	Ⓓ
21.	Ⓐ	Ⓑ	Ⓒ	Ⓓ	46.	Ⓐ	Ⓑ	Ⓒ	Ⓓ
22.	Ⓐ	Ⓑ	Ⓒ	Ⓓ	47.	Ⓐ	Ⓑ	Ⓒ	Ⓓ
23.	Ⓐ	Ⓑ	Ⓒ	Ⓓ	48.	Ⓐ	Ⓑ	Ⓒ	Ⓓ
24.	Ⓐ	Ⓑ	Ⓒ	Ⓓ	49.	Ⓐ	Ⓑ	Ⓒ	Ⓓ
25.	Ⓐ	Ⓑ	Ⓒ	Ⓓ	50.	Ⓐ	Ⓑ	Ⓒ	Ⓓ

V&S Publisher, Head Office: F-2/16 Ansari Road, Daryaganj, New Delhi-110002, Ph: 011-23240026-27, Email:info@vspublishers.com
Regional Office: 5-1-707/1, Brij Bhawan (Beside Central Bank of India Lane) Bank Street, Koti, Hyderabad-500 095, Ph: 040-24737290, Email: vspublishershyd@gmail.com
Branch: Jaywant Industrial Estate, 1st Floor–108, Tardeo Road Opposite Sobo Central Mall, Mumbai - 400 034, Ph: 022-23510736, Email: vspublishersmum@gmail.com

OMR ANSWER SHEET

1. NAME (IN ENGLISH CAPITAL LETTERS ONLY)

2. FATHER'S NAME (IN ENGLISH CAPITAL LETTERS ONLY)

Students must write and darken the respective circles completely for School Code, Class and Roll No. columns, othewise their Answer Sheets will not be evaluated.

3. SCHOOL CODE

School code columns with letters A–Z and digits 0–9.

4. % of Marks / Grade
In Last Class

Percentage OR Grade

Percentage digit columns 0–9; Grade columns A–J.

5. CLASS

Class columns with digits 0, 1, 2 and 4, 5, 6, 7, 8, 9, M, B.

6. ROLL NO.

Roll number columns with digits 0–9.

7. GENDER

MALE ○
FEMALE ○

8. STREAM
(Only for Class XI and XII Students)

MATHEMATICS ○
BIOLOGY ○
OTHERS ○

9. MARK YOUR ANSWERS WITH HB PENCIL/BALL POINT PEN (BLUE/BLACK)

1.	Ⓐ Ⓑ Ⓒ Ⓓ	26.	Ⓐ Ⓑ Ⓒ Ⓓ
2.	Ⓐ Ⓑ Ⓒ Ⓓ	27.	Ⓐ Ⓑ Ⓒ Ⓓ
3.	Ⓐ Ⓑ Ⓒ Ⓓ	28.	Ⓐ Ⓑ Ⓒ Ⓓ
4.	Ⓐ Ⓑ Ⓒ Ⓓ	29.	Ⓐ Ⓑ Ⓒ Ⓓ
5.	Ⓐ Ⓑ Ⓒ Ⓓ	30.	Ⓐ Ⓑ Ⓒ Ⓓ
6.	Ⓐ Ⓑ Ⓒ Ⓓ	31.	Ⓐ Ⓑ Ⓒ Ⓓ
7.	Ⓐ Ⓑ Ⓒ Ⓓ	32.	Ⓐ Ⓑ Ⓒ Ⓓ
8.	Ⓐ Ⓑ Ⓒ Ⓓ	33.	Ⓐ Ⓑ Ⓒ Ⓓ
9.	Ⓐ Ⓑ Ⓒ Ⓓ	34.	Ⓐ Ⓑ Ⓒ Ⓓ
10.	Ⓐ Ⓑ Ⓒ Ⓓ	35.	Ⓐ Ⓑ Ⓒ Ⓓ
11.	Ⓐ Ⓑ Ⓒ Ⓓ	36.	Ⓐ Ⓑ Ⓒ Ⓓ
12.	Ⓐ Ⓑ Ⓒ Ⓓ	37.	Ⓐ Ⓑ Ⓒ Ⓓ
13.	Ⓐ Ⓑ Ⓒ Ⓓ	38.	Ⓐ Ⓑ Ⓒ Ⓓ
14.	Ⓐ Ⓑ Ⓒ Ⓓ	39.	Ⓐ Ⓑ Ⓒ Ⓓ
15.	Ⓐ Ⓑ Ⓒ Ⓓ	40.	Ⓐ Ⓑ Ⓒ Ⓓ
16.	Ⓐ Ⓑ Ⓒ Ⓓ	41.	Ⓐ Ⓑ Ⓒ Ⓓ
17.	Ⓐ Ⓑ Ⓒ Ⓓ	42.	Ⓐ Ⓑ Ⓒ Ⓓ
18.	Ⓐ Ⓑ Ⓒ Ⓓ	43.	Ⓐ Ⓑ Ⓒ Ⓓ
19.	Ⓐ Ⓑ Ⓒ Ⓓ	44.	Ⓐ Ⓑ Ⓒ Ⓓ
20.	Ⓐ Ⓑ Ⓒ Ⓓ	45.	Ⓐ Ⓑ Ⓒ Ⓓ
21.	Ⓐ Ⓑ Ⓒ Ⓓ	46.	Ⓐ Ⓑ Ⓒ Ⓓ
22.	Ⓐ Ⓑ Ⓒ Ⓓ	47.	Ⓐ Ⓑ Ⓒ Ⓓ
23.	Ⓐ Ⓑ Ⓒ Ⓓ	48.	Ⓐ Ⓑ Ⓒ Ⓓ
24.	Ⓐ Ⓑ Ⓒ Ⓓ	49.	Ⓐ Ⓑ Ⓒ Ⓓ
25.	Ⓐ Ⓑ Ⓒ Ⓓ	50.	Ⓐ Ⓑ Ⓒ Ⓓ

V&S Publisher, Head Office: F-2/16 Ansari Road, Daryaganj, New Delhi-110002, Ph: 011-23240026-27, Email:info@vspublishers.com
Regional Office: 5-1-707/1, Brij Bhawan (Beside Central Bank of India Lane) Bank Street, Koti, Hyderabad-500 095, Ph: 040-24737290, Email: vspublishershyd@gmail.com
Branch: Jaywant Industrial Estate, 1st Floor–108, Tardeo Road Opposite Sobo Central Mall, Mumbai - 400 034, Ph: 022-23510736, Email: vspublishersmum@gmail.com

OMR ANSWER SHEET

1. NAME (IN ENGLISH CAPITAL LETTERS ONLY)

2. FATHER'S NAME (IN ENGLISH CAPITAL LETTERS ONLY)

Students must write and darken the respective circles completely for School Code, Class and Roll No. columns, othewise their Answer Sheets will not be evaluated.

3. SCHOOL CODE

A B C D E F G H I J K L M N O P Q R S T U V W X Y Z

0 1 2 3 4 5 6 7 8 9

4. % of Marks | Grade

In Last Class

Percentage OR Grade

0 1 2 3 4 5 6 7 8 9

A B C D E F G H I J

5. CLASS

0 1 2

6. ROLL NO.

0 1 2 3 4 5 6 7 8 9 M B

7. GENDER

MALE ○
FEMALE ○

8. STREAM
(Only for Class XI and XII Students)

MATHEMATICS ○
BIOLOGY ○
OTHERS ○

9. MARK YOUR ANSWERS WITH HB PENCIL/BALL POINT PEN (BLUE/BLACK)

No.					No.				
1.	Ⓐ	Ⓑ	Ⓒ	Ⓓ	26.	Ⓐ	Ⓑ	Ⓒ	Ⓓ
2.	Ⓐ	Ⓑ	Ⓒ	Ⓓ	27.	Ⓐ	Ⓑ	Ⓒ	Ⓓ
3.	Ⓐ	Ⓑ	Ⓒ	Ⓓ	28.	Ⓐ	Ⓑ	Ⓒ	Ⓓ
4.	Ⓐ	Ⓑ	Ⓒ	Ⓓ	29.	Ⓐ	Ⓑ	Ⓒ	Ⓓ
5.	Ⓐ	Ⓑ	Ⓒ	Ⓓ	30.	Ⓐ	Ⓑ	Ⓒ	Ⓓ
6.	Ⓐ	Ⓑ	Ⓒ	Ⓓ	31.	Ⓐ	Ⓑ	Ⓒ	Ⓓ
7.	Ⓐ	Ⓑ	Ⓒ	Ⓓ	32.	Ⓐ	Ⓑ	Ⓒ	Ⓓ
8.	Ⓐ	Ⓑ	Ⓒ	Ⓓ	33.	Ⓐ	Ⓑ	Ⓒ	Ⓓ
9.	Ⓐ	Ⓑ	Ⓒ	Ⓓ	34.	Ⓐ	Ⓑ	Ⓒ	Ⓓ
10.	Ⓐ	Ⓑ	Ⓒ	Ⓓ	35.	Ⓐ	Ⓑ	Ⓒ	Ⓓ
11.	Ⓐ	Ⓑ	Ⓒ	Ⓓ	36.	Ⓐ	Ⓑ	Ⓒ	Ⓓ
12.	Ⓐ	Ⓑ	Ⓒ	Ⓓ	37.	Ⓐ	Ⓑ	Ⓒ	Ⓓ
13.	Ⓐ	Ⓑ	Ⓒ	Ⓓ	38.	Ⓐ	Ⓑ	Ⓒ	Ⓓ
14.	Ⓐ	Ⓑ	Ⓒ	Ⓓ	39.	Ⓐ	Ⓑ	Ⓒ	Ⓓ
15.	Ⓐ	Ⓑ	Ⓒ	Ⓓ	40.	Ⓐ	Ⓑ	Ⓒ	Ⓓ
16.	Ⓐ	Ⓑ	Ⓒ	Ⓓ	41.	Ⓐ	Ⓑ	Ⓒ	Ⓓ
17.	Ⓐ	Ⓑ	Ⓒ	Ⓓ	42.	Ⓐ	Ⓑ	Ⓒ	Ⓓ
18.	Ⓐ	Ⓑ	Ⓒ	Ⓓ	43.	Ⓐ	Ⓑ	Ⓒ	Ⓓ
19.	Ⓐ	Ⓑ	Ⓒ	Ⓓ	44.	Ⓐ	Ⓑ	Ⓒ	Ⓓ
20.	Ⓐ	Ⓑ	Ⓒ	Ⓓ	45.	Ⓐ	Ⓑ	Ⓒ	Ⓓ
21.	Ⓐ	Ⓑ	Ⓒ	Ⓓ	46.	Ⓐ	Ⓑ	Ⓒ	Ⓓ
22.	Ⓐ	Ⓑ	Ⓒ	Ⓓ	47.	Ⓐ	Ⓑ	Ⓒ	Ⓓ
23.	Ⓐ	Ⓑ	Ⓒ	Ⓓ	48.	Ⓐ	Ⓑ	Ⓒ	Ⓓ
24.	Ⓐ	Ⓑ	Ⓒ	Ⓓ	49.	Ⓐ	Ⓑ	Ⓒ	Ⓓ
25.	Ⓐ	Ⓑ	Ⓒ	Ⓓ	50.	Ⓐ	Ⓑ	Ⓒ	Ⓓ

V&S Publisher, Head Office: F-2/16 Ansari Road, Daryaganj, New Delhi-110002, Ph: 011-23240026-27, Email:info@vspublishers.com
Regional Office: 5-1-707/1, Brij Bhawan (Beside Central Bank of India Lane) Bank Street, Koti, Hyderabad-500 095, Ph: 040-24737290, Email: vspublishershyd@gmail.com
Branch: Jaywant Industrial Estate, 1st Floor–108, Tardeo Road Opposite Sobo Central Mall, Mumbai - 400 034, Ph: 022-23510736, Email: vspublishersmum@gmail.com

OMR ANSWER SHEET

1. NAME (IN ENGLISH CAPITAL LETTERS ONLY)

2. FATHER'S NAME (IN ENGLISH CAPITAL LETTERS ONLY)

Students must write and darken the respective circles completely for School Code, Class and Roll No. columns, othewise their Answer Sheets will not be evaluated.

3. SCHOOL CODE

A B C D E F G H I J K L M N O P Q R S T U V W X Y Z
0 1 2 3 4 5 6 7 8 9

4. % of Marks | Grade

In Last Class

Percentage OR Grade

0 1 2 3 4 5 6 7 8 9
A B C D E F G H I J

5. CLASS

0 1 2 4 5 6 7 8 9 M B

6. ROLL NO.

0 1 2 3 4 5 6 7 8 9

7. GENDER

MALE ○
FEMALE ○

8. STREAM
(Only for Class XI and XII Students)

MATHEMATICS ○
BIOLOGY ○
OTHERS ○

9. MARK YOUR ANSWERS WITH HB PENCIL/BALL POINT PEN (BLUE/BLACK)

1.	A B C D	26.	A B C D
2.	A B C D	27.	A B C D
3.	A B C D	28.	A B C D
4.	A B C D	29.	A B C D
5.	A B C D	30.	A B C D
6.	A B C D	31.	A B C D
7.	A B C D	32.	A B C D
8.	A B C D	33.	A B C D
9.	A B C D	34.	A B C D
10.	A B C D	35.	A B C D
11.	A B C D	36.	A B C D
12.	A B C D	37.	A B C D
13.	A B C D	38.	A B C D
14.	A B C D	39.	A B C D
15.	A B C D	40.	A B C D
16.	A B C D	41.	A B C D
17.	A B C D	42.	A B C D
18.	A B C D	43.	A B C D
19.	A B C D	44.	A B C D
20.	A B C D	45.	A B C D
21.	A B C D	46.	A B C D
22.	A B C D	47.	A B C D
23.	A B C D	48.	A B C D
24.	A B C D	49.	A B C D
25.	A B C D	50.	A B C D

V&S Publisher, Head Office: F-2/16 Ansari Road, Daryaganj, New Delhi-110002, Ph: 011-23240026-27, Email:info@vspublishers.com
Regional Office: 5-1-707/1, Brij Bhawan (Beside Central Bank of India Lane) Bank Street, Koti, Hyderabad-500 095, Ph: 040-24737290, Email: vspublishershyd@gmail.com
Branch: Jaywant Industrial Estate, 1st Floor–108, Tardeo Road Opposite Sobo Central Mall, Mumbai - 400 034, Ph: 022-23510736, Email: vspublishersmum@gmail.com

OMR ANSWER SHEET

1. NAME (IN ENGLISH CAPITAL LETTERS ONLY)

2. FATHER'S NAME (IN ENGLISH CAPITAL LETTERS ONLY)

Students must write and darken the respective circles completely for School Code, Class and Roll No. columns, othewise their Answer Sheets will not be evaluated.

3. SCHOOL CODE

(A) (A) (0) (0) (0) (0)
(B) (B) (1) (1) (1) (1)
(C) (C) (2) (2) (2) (2)
(D) (D) (3) (3) (3) (3)
(E) (E) (4) (4) (4) (4)
(F) (F) (5) (5) (5) (5)
(G) (G) (6) (6) (6) (6)
(H) (H) (7) (7) (7) (7)
(I) (I) (8) (8) (8) (8)
(J) (J) (9) (9) (9) (9)
(K) (K)
(L) (L)
(M) (M)
(N) (N)
(O) (O)
(P) (P)
(Q) (Q)
(R) (R)
(S) (S)
(T) (T)
(U) (U)
(V) (V)
(W) (W)
(X) (X)
(Y) (Y)
(Z) (Z)

4. % of Marks | Grade
In Last Class

Percentage	OR	Grade

(0) (0) (0)   (A)
(1) (1) (1)   (B)
(2) (2) (2)   (C)
(3) (3) (3)   (D)
(4) (4) (4)   (E)
(5) (5) (5)   (F)
(6) (6) (6)   (G)
(7) (7) (7)   (H)
(8) (8) (8)   (I)
(9) (9) (9)   (J)

5. CLASS

(0) (0)
(1) (1)
(2) (2)
(4)
(5)
(6)
(7)
(8)
(9)
(M)
(B)

6. ROLL NO.

(0) (0) (0)
(1) (1) (1)
(2) (2) (2)
(3) (3)
(4) (4) (4)
(5) (5) (5)
(6) (6) (6)
(7) (7) (7)
(8) (8) (8)
(9) (9)

7. GENDER

MALE ○
FEMALE ○

8. STREAM
(Only for Class XI and XII Students)

MATHEMATICS ○
BIOLOGY ○
OTHERS ○

9. MARK YOUR ANSWERS WITH HB PENCIL/BALL POINT PEN (BLUE/BLACK)

1.	(A) (B) (C) (D)	26.	(A) (B) (C) (D)
2.	(A) (B) (C) (D)	27.	(A) (B) (C) (D)
3.	(A) (B) (C) (D)	28.	(A) (B) (C) (D)
4.	(A) (B) (C) (D)	29.	(A) (B) (C) (D)
5.	(A) (B) (C) (D)	30.	(A) (B) (C) (D)
6.	(A) (B) (C) (D)	31.	(A) (B) (C) (D)
7.	(A) (B) (C) (D)	32.	(A) (B) (C) (D)
8.	(A) (B) (C) (D)	33.	(A) (B) (C) (D)
9.	(A) (B) (C) (D)	34.	(A) (B) (C) (D)
10.	(A) (B) (C) (D)	35.	(A) (B) (C) (D)
11.	(A) (B) (C) (D)	36.	(A) (B) (C) (D)
12.	(A) (B) (C) (D)	37.	(A) (B) (C) (D)
13.	(A) (B) (C) (D)	38.	(A) (B) (C) (D)
14.	(A) (B) (C) (D)	39.	(A) (B) (C) (D)
15.	(A) (B) (C) (D)	40.	(A) (B) (C) (D)
16.	(A) (B) (C) (D)	41.	(A) (B) (C) (D)
17.	(A) (B) (C) (D)	42.	(A) (B) (C) (D)
18.	(A) (B) (C) (D)	43.	(A) (B) (C) (D)
19.	(A) (B) (C) (D)	44.	(A) (B) (C) (D)
20.	(A) (B) (C) (D)	45.	(A) (B) (C) (D)
21.	(A) (B) (C) (D)	46.	(A) (B) (C) (D)
22.	(A) (B) (C) (D)	47.	(A) (B) (C) (D)
23.	(A) (B) (C) (D)	48.	(A) (B) (C) (D)
24.	(A) (B) (C) (D)	49.	(A) (B) (C) (D)
25.	(A) (B) (C) (D)	50.	(A) (B) (C) (D)

V&S Publisher, Head Office: F-2/16 Ansari Road, Daryaganj, New Delhi-110002, Ph: 011-23240026-27, Email:info@vspublishers.com
Regional Office: 5-1-707/1, Brij Bhawan (Beside Central Bank of India Lane) Bank Street, Koti, Hyderabad-500 095, Ph: 040-24737290, Email: vspublishershyd@gmail.com
Branch: Jaywant Industrial Estate, 1st Floor–108, Tardeo Road Opposite Sobo Central Mall, Mumbai - 400 034, Ph: 022-23510736, Email: vspublishersmum@gmail.com